MONTVALE PUBLIC LIBRARY

MONTVALE PUBLIC LIBRARY, NJ

W9-ABV-010

ON LINE

3 9125 05034950 5

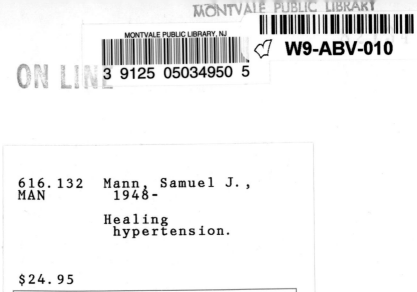

616.132   Mann, Samuel J.,
MAN   1948-

          Healing
           hypertension.

$24.95

DATE			

BAKER & TAYLOR

Healing Hypertension

Uncovering the Secret Power
of Your Hidden Emotions

Samuel J. Mann, M.D.

John Wiley & Sons, Inc.

New York • Chichester • Weinheim • Brisbane • Singapore • Toronto

This book is printed on acid-free paper. ∞

Copyright © 1999 by Samuel J. Mann. All rights reserved.

Published simultaneously in Canada

No part of this publication may be reproduced, stored in a retrieval system or transmitted in any form or by any means, electronic, mechanical, photocopying, recording, scanning or otherwise, except as permitted under Section 107 or 108 of the 1976 United States Copyright Act, without either the prior written permission of the Publisher, or authorization through payment of the appropriate per-copy fee to the Copyright Clearance Center, 222 Rosewood Drive, Danvers, MA 01923, (978) 750-8400, fax (978) 750-4744. Requests to the Publisher for permission should be addressed to the Permissions Department, John Wiley & Sons, Inc., 605 Third Avenue, New York, NY 10158-0012, (212) 850-6011, fax (212) 850-6008, E-Mail: PERMREQ@WILEY.COM.

This publication is designed to provide accurate and authoritative information in regard to the subject matter covered. It is sold with the understanding that the publisher is not engaged in rendering professional services. If professional advice or other expert assistance is required, the services of a competent professional person should be sought.

Library of Congress Cataloging-in-Publication Data:

Mann, Samuel J.
    Healing hypertension : uncovering the secret power of your
hidden emotions / Samuel J. Mann.
        p.   cm.
    Includes bibliographical references and index.
    ISBN 0-471-17547-1 (cloth : alk. paper)
    1. Hypertension—Popular works. 2. Hypertension—Psychosomatic aspects. 3. Hypertension—Etiology.   I. Title.
    RC685.H8M283   1999
    616.1′32—dc21   98-17434

Printed in the United States of America

10 9 8 7 6 5 4 3 2 1

To my wife, Maureen, to David,
and to Sammy, with all my love.

MONTVALE PUBLIC LIBRARY

Contents

PART 2: *Solving the Mind–Body Mystery*

Acknowledgments

I had no interest in writing throughout my years of school. I developed no writing skills and the thought of writing a book never occurred to me. However, on a flight from Washington, D.C., to New York in 1990, a woman sitting next to me suggested that I ought to write one. The moment she suggested it, I knew I would write it, no matter what it took, even though I knew nothing about writing a book. I am grateful, first and foremost, to the human mind that gives us the capacity to do things we might never have dreamed of, and to will us to do them even when the odds seem insurmountable. I am grateful for the life experiences, good and bad, the wise words I have read and heard, the people who have entered my life, and the passion with which we are all endowed that made this book possible.

I am grateful for the good fortune to have met everyone I needed to in order to write the book. I start out with my wife, Maureen, who has understood my barriers to relationship (and I hers) as we build our partnership in life. She held things together while I disappeared into the otherworld of extended focus on the book. I also want to thank my son David who at his tender age respected my need to ration my time with him more than I would have liked.

I am grateful to my parents and sister. I could not have written this book without the childhood years I spent with them, and the good and bad experiences of those years. They gave me all they could.

The book is a collaborative effort with my patients. Together we were dissatisfied with the diagnosis of "essential" hypertension. Together we sought the reasons and shared the struggle to understand the way in which mind and body were affecting each other. It was a bumpy path but one that led eventually to an understanding that made sense and offered a better way to approach treatment.

Charles Bloom stands big in my life. I have enjoyed a succession of relationships with Charlie. He has been healer, mentor, colleague, and friend. He helped me open the door to a very different life from the one I had known. His encouragement and selfless support helped me through periods of great doubt, and rekindled my passion whenever it was at low ebb. I can never adequately express my gratitude or understand the good fortune that brought Charlie into my life.

Sukie Miller entered my life just when I needed her and helped me to understand things that I had never realized I needed to understand. She became the best friend I ever had as a child.

I could never have learned what I have learned about hypertension without the opportunities given me by Dr. John Laragh, my mentor for over a decade at the Hypertension Center, which he founded. Dr. Laragh is a pioneer in the field of hypertension and of the philosophy of seeking the medication that matches the mechanism causing a person's hypertension. I would never have had the opportunity to see the thousands of patients I have seen and to learn from them without the institution that he created. We agreed on many things and disagreed on a few, and had our good times and bad ones. My gratitude will not diminish over time.

I want to thank John Wiley and Sons, Inc., for taking on my proposal and having the confidence that I could write the book. My editor, Judith McCarthy, had the subtle sense of knowing how to criticize without my knowing that I was being criticized. It was invaluable to a novice writer. I also want to thank my agent, Jean Naggar, who believed in my ideas, stayed the course with me, and skillfully steered the proposal to the right placement. I also owe a debt to the editors who read and rejected my first proposal four years ago. They knew better than I that I was not ready at the time. The system worked.

I want to thank Howard Greenwald, Frank Banton, and Paul Pendorf for kindly reading the manuscript, and Charles Bloom, Susan Mintzer, Mark Kuras, and Barbara Barak for their highly professional critiques of the book's concepts.

I shared my first papers on the mind–body relationship of hypertension with my Uncle Jimmy (Dr. James Mann), who died in 1996. I would have loved to have shared the satisfaction of the publication of this book with him.

I want to thank Dr. Mutya San Agustin for her support and friendship over the years, and Dr. Robert Allan, who stimulated me to critically examine my views. Dr. Nathan Schwartz-Salant helped me in refining psychological concepts. Dr. Jim Strain's enthusiastic encouragement was very important to me. Discussing ideas with Dr. Ron Sunshine was helpful to me. Dr. Phyllis August, successor to Dr. Laragh as head of the Hypertension Center, allowed me the flexibility without which I could not have completed the book.

I am grateful to the Sielecky family and to Ronald Stanton, whose generous support for my research and learning process seemed to come at exactly the right time.

My friendships with Jeff Waldhuter and Benny Barak have been a bulwark through good and bad times. I also want to thank Judy Kreuter, whose home I was able to sneak away to for undisturbed trysts with my laptop.

The Sabbath was a great friend, which cost me a day of work each week, but probably helped me finish sooner without experiencing writer's block.

I WILL NEVER UNDERSTAND the mysterious ways in which the mind works to lead us to find the meaning in our lives. While I can take credit for the perseverance and hours of work I put into the book, I can merely acknowledge the forces within us that guide us and that have guided me in my writing.

Introduction

FOR THE PAST FIFTEEN YEARS I have had the unique opportunity of evaluating and treating thousands of people with hypertension—high blood pressure—at the Hypertension Center of the New York Hospital–Cornell Medical Center. Based on this experience, I have acquired an understanding that I believe can help you finally make sense of your hypertension. This book explains how I came to this understanding and how it can change the way you approach your high blood pressure.

My Path to Understanding Hypertension

As a specialist treating hypertension, prescribing medications and manipulating their dosage and combinations became second nature to me long ago. However, the mystery of why people develop hypertension has always intrigued me. It has been of even greater concern to my patients, who regularly ask me the same question: "*Why* do I have hypertension?" It is amazing that after decades of research over 95 percent of people with hypertension are still labeled as having *essential hypertension,* meaning the cause is unknown.

I don't accept this conclusion. I believe it is possible to make sense of hypertension most of the time and to pursue the most appropriate and effective individual treatment depending on the cause. *Healing Hypertension* is dedicated to this belief.

WHEN I DECIDED to specialize in hypertension, my career goal was to combine clinical practice and research. Questions that arose while I was seeing patients stimulated my research goals. Over the years I published articles in leading medical and hypertension journals, attended meetings of hypertension societies, and mingled with researchers from around the world to debate the meaning of findings in basic science and clinical research.

However, despite impressive advances in scientific knowledge about essential hypertension, I still could not tell many of my patients why they had the condition. I began to realize that refinement of knowledge about the physical body, from organ systems to cells to genes, would probably never enable doctors to explain why a person whose blood pressure was perfectly normal five years ago now has rip-roaring hypertension for no obvious reason.

I also became familiar with the many studies focused on the mind–body connection of hypertension. At first I did not have any particular interest in this area. If anything, like many of my colleagues, I scoffed at researchers who focused on the interaction between emotional stress and high blood pressure. I was also oblivious to the effects on our health of what I will call "hidden" emotions. My overall view was that mind–body research was pretty much a waste of time.

It is in spite of this orientation, or ironically because of it, that I ended up writing *Healing Hypertension*. I understand why people are reluctant to consider the effect of hidden emotions on their physical health because I felt the same way. It took very compelling observations to change my views.

IN MY WORK WITH PATIENTS I began to notice a pattern that contradicted the usual view of the link between stress and hypertension. Even patients with severe hypertension did not seem more emotionally distressed than others. If anything, they seemed less distressed. Their high blood pressure appeared to be more related to what they did *not* seem to be feeling than to what they *were* feeling.

I was often surprised when I noticed that many very anxious people who came to me already diagnosed as having hypertension did not truly have the condition and often didn't need the medication they were taking. I began to doubt that hypertension usually was a disease of *hyper* people and found that most studies supported my suspicions.

When I began to find a link between hypertension and hidden emotions, I assumed at first that this link was present only in the rare person. As time went on, I began to observe it in a much larger proportion of my patients. I learned more about the subtleties and masks people utilized to hide these emotions from me, from others, and mostly from themselves. I began to listen more carefully and pay more attention to what my patients were *not* telling me, particularly those with severe or difficult-to-control hypertension or other unexplained physical problems. I learned that high blood pressure was linked to hidden emotions in some people but not others. In time I learned how to tell in whom it was, and in whom it was not.

I questioned my evolving understanding again and again. I was concerned that I was allowing myself to be misled by coincidences. These concerns subsided as continued observations strengthened my evolving beliefs. When I began to see hypertension disappear in patients who gained awareness of hidden emotions, I became further convinced.

My beliefs were reinforced by changes in my own life that similarly resulted from uncovering emotions I had never suspected I harbored. This healing effect contributed greatly toward my understanding of the role of these emotions in hypertension.

WHEN I ENTERED MY LATE THIRTIES, I was unmarried. My relationships had followed a repetitive pattern. I would very much like a woman and enjoy being with her, but then I would decide I didn't love her and would eventually end the relationship. I did not understand why the same feeling always recurred. I didn't love her. I became concerned that time was threatening to preclude marriage and family, and I began to look into the reasons for my behavior pattern.

Almost incidentally during this process, I began to think more about Mary, an elderly woman who had been a live-in baby-sitter for my sister and me during our early childhood. She had always been very loving and available. She had no family of her own and we had become her family. She loved my sister and me like a grandmother. She had lived with us as far back as I could remember and I always saw her as part of our family.

Mary developed metastatic breast cancer when I was nine. I clearly remembered her final bedridden weeks. I would return home from school and run upstairs to her room to talk with her. One day, I came home and ran up to her room, but found it empty. She had died.

In those days children did not go to funerals, and in my home, as in many homes, death was not discussed with children. Mary was rarely mentioned after her death. I remember being teary for a few nights while alone in my bed, but I didn't or couldn't share my grief with anyone. From that point on, I recalled Mary as the woman who had lived with us, but not as someone I had loved.

THINKING ABOUT MARY AGAIN for the first time in decades, I felt an urge to light a candle in her memory—something I had never done. For months I did not act on this urge, but it remained. I finally pledged to myself that I would do so before my next birthday. It arrived, and still I had not acted. Finally, after two sleepless nights, I realized I had no choice.

Mary was Catholic, so I went to St. Patrick's Cathedral after work, lit a candle, sat down, and a dam burst. I found myself flooded with grief. I felt as if Mary had just died two or three weeks ago, not thirty years ago. In my grief I was able to talk to her, and tell her things that I was incapable of telling her when I was nine—that I loved her and that she had been very important to me, that I wished I had told her how I felt so that she could have known and enjoyed feeling loved.

I also understood why for all those years I didn't realize that I had loved her. Losing her had been too painful to tolerate by myself at that age. Instead I told myself I didn't love her. Therefore, I didn't feel the pain of losing her.

I had never let go of Mary. I had never grieved. I had never fully accepted my love for her and the loss of that love. I realized why a person who has not accepted a loss, such as that of a loved spouse, has difficulty moving on to marry again. In that moment I sensed that I had not been free to love another woman.

I left the church a million pounds lighter. I felt relieved of a huge burden I never knew I had been carrying within me. I realized this was only one piece of my healing process. However, eight months later—perhaps by coincidence, perhaps not—I met my future wife.

NO TEXTBOOK could ever enable me to understand as clearly as my own experience that we can harbor extremely painful emotions and not know it. Or that these emotions survive unchanged, independent of time, and affect us even decades later.

About the Book

I will be covering a few central concepts in *Healing Hypertension:*

1. The tendency of blood pressure to fluctuate often causes confusion about who does and who does not truly have hypertension. This has led to the overdiagnosis and unnecessary treatment of millions of people. You will find out how to tell if you truly have hypertension and whether or not you need medication.

2. The focus in research on the emotional distress people feel has not adequately clarified the mind–body link of hypertension. Getting angry or tense can undoubtedly elevate your blood pressure for that moment, but it does not cause hypertension. Reining in your emotions is not the path to curing your hypertension.

3. It is our hidden emotions, the emotions we do not feel, that lead to hypertension and many other unexplained physical disorders. Looking at hypertension this way, you can make sense of it and discover a path toward healing.

4. Becoming aware of our hidden emotions and dealing with them can enable both physical and emotional healing. It is not easy, but the good news is that most of us are more capable than we think we are.

5. Finally, if you have hypertension and need medication to control it, knowledge of whether or not hidden emotions are playing a role can help your physician, in partnership with you, to select the right drug for you, by matching the drug to the cause of your hypertension.

I want to emphasize strongly that hypertension can be caused by a number of factors, alone or in combination. In many people, hypertension is driven mainly by hidden emotions. In many others it is not, and such factors as genetics, obesity, and salt consumption are more important. I shall explain how you can tell whether hidden emotions are relevant to your hypertension. It makes no sense to focus on them if your hypertension is mainly genetic. However, if hidden emotions are involved, it is important to recognize the opportunity for both physical and emotional healing.

Learning from the Laboratory and from Life

Many scientific articles have been written about emotions and hypertension. Their results are not consistent and they provide support for any and every point of view. I could easily fill this book with a presentation and critique of this mammoth literature, but given its inconsistency I have chosen to present that literature succinctly. Where possible, I cite reviews that summarize the findings of many studies.

I have also chosen to avoid complicated medical or psychological jargon as much as possible in the hope that everyone who reads this book will be able to understand the ideas presented in it.

IT IS NOT AN ACCIDENT that this book was written by a physician and not by a psychologist. Hypertension is a medical condition. It is treated by physicians, not psychologists. As a specialist at the Hypertension Center, I had the opportunity to see and learn from thousands of patients.

The insight that I have accumulated did not arise primarily from observations in laboratory experiments. It arose largely from the unique experience of talking one-on-one with thousands of people with hypertension and merging knowledge gained from this experience with my medical knowledge and training.

I want to emphasize that my observations concerning hidden emotions do not disagree with what medical and psychological studies have reported. They are wholly consistent with what science has taught us about hypertension, but they go further in helping to fill in the large persisting gap in our understanding of essential hypertension.

I have learned a great deal from the studies I have read. However, I have learned far more from people and their stories than from reading about their reactions to artificial stressors in the laboratory. I believe it is time to return to observing and listening to people rather than relying solely on research dominated by number crunching and complex statistical analyses that provides data that are largely irrelevant to real patients in doctors' offices.

The stories I will share do not represent rare cases. They are all from the practice of a single physician and they are the kinds of cases I see again and again. Most of my patients have come to me because of the distinguished medical reputation of the Hypertension Center. They are not a select group specifically oriented to mind–body approaches. Thus, I am confident you will find my observations relevant to your search for an understanding of your hypertension.

In relating patients' stories, I have changed some of the personal details to protect their privacy. In addition, some of the case histories represent a composite of patients with similar stories. However, I have taken great care to ensure that the essence of their stories is preserved.

We learn most from stories of people like ourselves. You might see a resemblance between your own story and one of the many stories I share in the book. If so, it is my hope that this will help open your path to insight and healing.

THIS BOOK PRESENTS my journey of discovery. It describes what my patients have taught me. I have tried to present my understanding in the way in which it unfolded to me. I invite you to join me on that journey.

Hypertension:
The Great Mystery

Unearthing the Causes of Hypertension

Y OU ARE IN YOUR FORTIES. You are slim and go to the gym four times a week. You get along with your spouse and you have a good job.

You have one medical problem: high blood pressure. Tests could not find a cause for it, and, by default, like 95 percent or more of people with high blood pressure, you are considered to have "essential hypertension." You have been told you will have to take pills, possibly for the rest of your life. You might go to another doctor who will repeat some of the tests or manipulate the medications, but the end result will be the same: You have hypertension and no one can tell you why.

Scenarios like this are played out regularly in physicians' offices. No one can tell you why you have hypertension. Even people with severe hypertension arrive at this same dead end: pills and no explanation. Even worse, you may have been led to believe that this condition is your own fault, because you are too "hyper."

FIFTY MILLION AMERICANS have hypertension. It is responsible for more visits to the doctor than any other medical condition. As the leading risk factor for strokes and a leading risk factor for heart attacks, it is a major health concern. Billions of dollars are spent each year on drugs, doctor visits, and research. Yet, in case after case, the cause is still considered a mystery. My experience argues that this is wrong, that often we *can* understand why you have hypertension, and sometimes we can even cure it.

What Is Hypertension?

Hypertension, also known as high blood pressure, is a persisting elevation of the pressure of the blood circulating in the arteries throughout the body. Over time, it causes damage to the arteries and to organs that receive blood through them. Ultimately it leads to an increased risk of cardiovascular events such as strokes and heart attacks, and, in severe cases, to heart and/or kidney failure. The more severe the hypertension, the sooner and more likely the complications.

Hypertension is unlikely to cause physical symptoms that warn of its presence unless it is very severe. Most people who have hypertension do not have headaches or feel a pressure in their head or feel dizzy. Most feel perfectly well. This is why hypertension has been called the "silent time bomb." Generally it is found only by measuring the blood pressure.

The components of the blood pressure measurement are the systolic and diastolic pressures, which represent the rise and fall of blood pressure associated with each heartbeat. Just as a mechanical pump pushes fluid into a system of pipes, the heart pumps blood into the aorta and the arteries to circulate oxygen and nutrients throughout the body. The forceful contraction of the heart pushes blood forward and raises the pressure. This peak pressure is called the systolic pressure. Between heartbeats, the pressure in the arterial system falls to the level known as the diastolic pressure.

Blood pressure is typically recorded as the systolic pressure over the diastolic pressure. An example of a normal reading would be 120/80, read as "120 over 80." The number 120 represents 120 millimeters of mercury, as explained below.

Since blood pressure fluctuates from moment to moment, I usually check a patient's blood pressure several times over a minute or so, and record it either as an average value or as the range of the readings I have obtained. For example, if the systolic pressure varied between 120 and 130, and the diastolic between 75 and 85, I would record it as 120–130/75–85.

Blood pressure is measured by placing a cuff around the upper arm and inflating it with air, causing the cuff to tighten around the arm. The pressure with which it is compressing the arm is measured as the millimeters of height it raises a column of mercury, as depicted in Figure 1.1.

The cuff is inflated to a pressure higher than the blood pressure, at which point it will completely block the flow of blood through the brachial artery, the main artery in the arm. Then the cuff is slowly deflated and the column of mercury begins to fall. The cuff pressure at which blood begins to resume flowing through the artery with each heartbeat is detected by the appearance of a sound with each heartbeat, called a *Korotkoff sound*. The sound is caused by the turbulence of blood flowing through the now partially open artery. The height of the mercury column when these sounds first appear is called the systolic pressure.

As the cuff deflation continues, and the pressure compressing the arm and the artery falls further, it impedes the flow of blood less and less. Finally, when blood flow is completely unimpeded, the turbulence ceases and the sounds disappear. The height of the mercury column when the sounds disappear is called the diastolic pressure.

OUR BLOOD PRESSURE VARIES from moment to moment. If we lift a heavy package or rush down the street or get really angry, it increases. If we relax and do nothing, it falls. As reviewed in the recent report of the Joint National Committee on Prevention, Detection, Evaluation and Treatment of High Blood Pressure (1997), or JNCVI, hypertension is diagnosed when your blood pressure averages above 140/90 while you are sitting quietly in your doctor's office. At home, your blood pressure is considered elevated if readings average above 130–135/85.

Hypertension is classified as mild, moderate, or severe, or more recently, according to the JNCVI, as Stage 1, 2, or 3, based

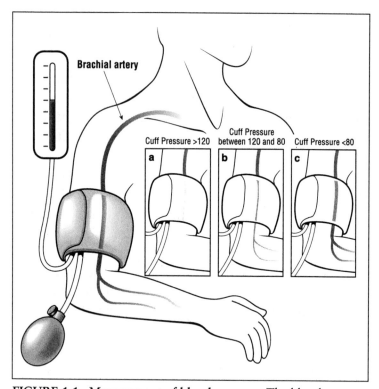

FIGURE 1.1. **Measurement of blood pressure.** The blood pressure cuff is inflated until it pushes the mercury column above the systolic pressure. It compresses the arm sufficiently to collapse and stop the flow of blood through the brachial artery, the main artery of the arm (a). As the cuff is deflated, blood flow will resume at the systolic pressure, which is 120 in this example (b). However, the persisting partial compression of the artery will cause turbulence of blood flow, producing the sounds heard through the stethoscope. At the diastolic pressure (c), the turbulence and sounds disappear as unimpeded blood flow resumes.

on the height of the blood pressure. Table 1 shows the percentage of people with hypertension who fall into each category. The risk of suffering complications from hypertension is proportional to your usual blood pressure level. Therefore, there is no reason to believe that your risk at 141/91, which is considered to be in the hypertensive range, differs much from the risk at 139/89, which is

TABLE 1: Classification of Individuals with Essential Hypertension

Hypertension Category	Systolic		Diastolic	Percent
Mild (Stage 1)	140–159	or	90–99	21
Moderate (Stage 2)	160–179	or	100–109	35
Severe (Stage 3)	Above 180	or	Above 110	44

Data obtained from the "Fifth Joint National Committee Report on the Detection, Evaluation and Treatment of High Blood Pressure" (Pogue et al., 1996).

not. Even so, if your readings approach 140/90, measures to reduce your blood pressure are worthwhile.

Our blood pressure level is determined by the force of contraction of the heart muscle, the volume of blood circulating within the arteries, and the state of contraction or relaxation of the arteries. These mechanisms are more thoroughly described in Chapter 13. As reviewed by Norman Kaplan in his textbook, *Clinical Hypertension*, it is believed that roughly 30 to 50 percent of hypertension is governed by genetic factors. The rest is governed by lifestyle factors such as weight, diet, emotions, alcohol consumption, and exercise. Recent reports also suggest that sleep apnea, a disorder marked by irregular breathing patterns during sleep, may be an important contributor to hypertension (see D. S. Silverberg, 1997). In any individual, hypertension may result primarily from either genetic or lifestyle factors, or a combination of both.

The Mind–Body Connection

If there ever was a condition believed to be tied to emotions and stress, it is hypertension. Yet surprisingly, decades of research have not shown that the emotional distress we feel is a major cause of hypertension or that relaxation techniques to reduce that distress can eliminate it. Contrary to popular expectations, research has not strongly supported the notion that people who have hypertension feel more tense or angry, or are under more stress, than people who don't.

In my experience as a physician specializing in the treatment of hypertension, I find the same thing. Most patients with hypertension, even if it is severe, do not claim to be particularly tense or angry. This seems very hard to believe. When I meet people socially and mention my specialty, many tell me they are "hypertense," (a word that does not exist, by the way), or say, "Boy, do *I* need to see you." Living in New York City, I hear this all the time, yet study results do not support this popular view of the mind–body relationship in hypertension.

However, my experience treating thousands of people with high blood pressure tells me there is a crucial connection with emotions, but one that is very different from what most people believe. It tells me that the emotions we feel usually have less to do with hypertension than do the emotions we harbor but *don't* feel and often don't even know exist within us. I believe this view offers an explanation for hypertension where traditional views have failed and offers an approach to treatment that can lead to both physical and emotional healing. It enables some people to get off medication and provides a rationale for selecting the right antihypertensive drug for those who need drug treatment.

Emotions Are Not Always the Cause of Hypertension

I see many patients in whom emotions play a major role in causing hypertension and many others in whom they do not. Thus, I believe it is wrong to say that all hypertension is caused by emotions, as some mind–body practitioners might suggest, or to recommend emotion-based treatment for everyone who has high blood pressure.

It would be just as wrong to say that hypertension is related to emotions in no one and that emotional factors should be ignored, as many physicians and medical researchers might say. I have personally seen hypertension improve in many patients when its emotional basis was correctly identified and addressed.

Whether your hypertension is related to emotions or not, I believe *Healing Hypertension* can help you better understand both its origin and its treatment. As I'll discuss, there are clues that can clarify whether your hypertension is related to hidden emotions. These clues are then useful both in selecting the right antihypertensive drugs and in determining whether to consider emotion-based therapy.

If emotional factors are contributing to your hypertension, I hope to clarify how blocking your emotions has worked to protect you but has also contributed to your condition. With this understanding, a path to healing is available if you choose it.

The Link between Hidden Emotions and Health in Other Conditions

Despite the explosion in medical knowledge in recent decades, the causes of many medical conditions, such as irritable bowel syndrome, colitis, chronic fatigue syndrome, fibromyalgia, and migraine, remain a mystery. Researchers have discovered biochemical abnormalities related to some of these conditions and drugs have been developed to address some of them. However, the causes of those abnormalities remain unknown. Studies of the emotional distress people feel have also failed to clarify their origin.

Medications sometimes help control the above conditions and sometimes don't. However, one thing the pills cannot do is cure them.

Aside from these conditions, many people suffer from a variety of unexplained physical symptoms. In a study by Kurt Kroenke reported in the *American Journal of Medicine* in 1989, an explanation could not be found 74 percent of the time when people sought medical attention for physical symptoms such as chest pain, fatigue, dizziness, headaches, insomnia, and weight loss. In such ailments the role of hidden emotions is widely ignored. If you suffer from any of these conditions, I hope you will consider the relevance of the lessons I have learned from people with hypertension.

The Shortcomings of Medication

The goal of treating hypertension is to lower blood pressure to normal and to prevent its cardiovascular complications. Ideally, we would like to accomplish this goal with medications that address the cause of the hypertension, are inexpensive, have no side effects, and always work. If we had achieved these goals, there would be no reason to consider alternative methods of treatment.

However, we have not achieved these goals. Medications do not always work, they are usually expensive, and they often cause side effects. Many people either cannot remember to take pills every day or just don't want to. No one is particularly thrilled about taking pills every day for the rest of his life.

The shortcomings of treatment are evident in the findings of the National Health and Nutritional Examination survey, reported by Vicki Burt in the journal *Hypertension* in 1995. It found that only 69 percent of people with hypertension were aware of their condition and that it was controlled (blood pressure below 140/90) in only 27 percent. There is no question that the medication available today is more effective and has far fewer side effects than the medication available twenty years ago. However, it is also clear that we have far to go before we eliminate the health problems that result from hypertension.

Finally, as elegantly discussed by Stevo Julius in the journal *Hypertension* in 1993, the increased activation of the sympathetic nervous system that underlies hypertension in many people, and that is the likely link between emotions and hypertension, has many harmful effects other than just high blood pressure. It increases our coronary risk by altering hormone levels, blood clotting, and blood vessels through mechanisms other than hypertension. Lowering the blood pressure with pills does not eliminate these effects, which might explain why even perfect blood pressure control will not completely eliminate the excess risk of coronary disease associated with hypertension.

An Epidemic of Overdiagnosis

The diagnosis of hypertension is not always clear-cut. It is not like cancer, where usually someone either has it or doesn't. In many people, the systolic blood pressure is only minimally elevated, or might fluctuate above and below 140. In others, the blood pressure is elevated only while it is being measured and is normal at all other times.

These problems have led to an epidemic of overdiagnosis and unnecessary treatment for millions who do not truly have hypertension. As I shall discuss, there is considerable evidence that at least a quarter of those diagnosed with hypertension do not have it and do not require treatment. If you are in this category, I hope the book will help you get off unneeded medication and will reduce your concern that you are at high risk for suffering a stroke.

In order to understand the relationship between hidden emotions and hypertension, we must first be clear as to who truly has hypertension and who does not. I shall begin by first addressing this important issue.

Do You Really Have Hypertension?

2

ALONG WITH the growing general awareness of hypertension, there has also been an epidemic of overdiagnosis. In this chapter I shall discuss the reasons for this and describe how you can tell whether you really have hypertension.

The Alerting Reaction and White Coat Hypertension

For many people, a blood pressure check has become a stressful event. Some are afraid that they are at risk of suffering a sudden stroke, particularly if a parent died of a complication of hypertension. Sometimes it is frightening simply because of what we read about hypertension. The designation "silent time bomb" does not exactly calm people who have been told that their blood pressure is high. In many people, such fears contribute to the temporary elevation of blood pressure at the time of measurement, a phenomenon termed an "alerting response," which can lead to a misdiagnosis of hypertension.

I would suspect that the alerting response happened less often when the average person knew little about hypertension. The media attention of the past few decades has converted the moment of blood pressure measurement into a moment of truth, an emotional event whose effect on the measurement is not neutral.

A study reported by Morten Rostrup in the *American Journal of Hypertension* in 1990 documents this rather dramatically. He found that people who were told that their blood pressure was elevated had a higher reading at their next visit than people who were told nothing. Isaac Amigo, in a study published in the *Journal of Hypertension* in 1993, similarly found that if he told subjects their blood pressure was high, their readings climbed 4 millimeters by the next visit. If he told them their blood pressure was fine, it fell 8 millimeters. In the same way, in many people, once a single elevated reading introduces fear, all further readings can be elevated.

Many patients with the mildest of hypertension believe they are at high risk of having a stroke at any moment. However, with rare exceptions, your risk of stroke increases only after many years of hypertension. Another popular misconception is that a brief increase in blood pressure, for example, to a systolic pressure above 200 or a diastolic pressure above 120, can cause a sudden stroke. Such an occurrence is extremely rare.

Weight lifters, for example, can have readings as high as 230/140 while lifting weights, even if at other times their blood pressure is perfectly normal (see J. Sullivan, 1992). Yet people do not suffer strokes while lifting weights.

Some people feel reassured only when they are placed on medication. Once treated and feeling reassured, their blood pressure of course falls, confirming to them that they needed the medication. Not surprisingly, if you begin medication and your blood pressure returns to normal, both you and your physician will conclude that the medicine is working well, rather than considering that you might not have had hypertension in the first place. Maybe this is why, in almost every study reported, one of every three people with elevated blood pressure readings responds to a mere placebo—a dummy pill.

The temporary rise in blood pressure caused by nervousness during its measurement has fueled the belief that anxiety is a frequent cause of hypertension. Further validating this myth, learning how to relax during the measurement lowers the readings. This suggests to people that anxiety caused their hypertension and that treating the anxiety was the cure, when it was actually only the alerting reaction during measurement that was affected.

Many people have an extremely elevated blood pressure in the physician's office and yet a very normal blood pressure at home. Many patients tell me that the blood pressure apparatus they use at home must be inaccurate because the readings are so good. Some even throw out the machine!

Many studies have compared readings obtained at the physician's office with readings obtained at home. These studies, such as one published by Thomas Pickering in 1988, uniformly reveal that about 20 to 25 percent of people diagnosed as having hypertension based on physician readings have normal blood pressure readings at home. Most studies show that these patients, who have what is called "white coat hypertension," bear a much lower risk than patients whose blood pressure is also elevated at home.

I often see patients with mildly elevated readings who I suspect do not have hypertension. I tell them that I am not certain that they have hypertension, and that if they do, it is mild and they are not at high risk of having a stroke. In many instances this reassurance alone has led to lower readings at follow-up visits. If they are on medication, I can often discontinue it, although I follow their blood pressure carefully. Others, whose readings in my office remain elevated, might still have white coat hypertension, and I recommend monitoring their blood pressure outside my office, as described below.

Just to complicate the picture a little further, many people who have white coat hypertension feel perfectly calm while their blood pressure is soaring during its measurement. Despite what you might think, you can have white coat hypertension no matter how you feel during the measurement.

Sometimes, when I suspect white coat hypertension, I ask a nurse to check a patient's blood pressure. However, I have come to rely more and more on the readings patients obtain at home. These readings are usually very representative of their true blood pressure, although sometimes even these readings must be interpreted with caution.

▶ Charlie, thirty-nine, an attorney, had first been told of elevated blood pressure readings when he was sixteen. He checks his blood pressure regularly at home and has reported to me that, on average, it is slightly elevated, running about 135/95. Charlie is thin and has no family history of hypertension. In my office, his blood pressure was 110–120/88. I told him I did not think he had hypertension.

Over the next four months, his blood pressure at home was consistently 125/85, lower than it had been in years. There was no other change to account for the improvement in his blood pressure, other than my telling him I did not think he had hypertension. ◀

Your concern can sometimes affect your blood pressure readings even at home. If you are extremely nervous when you check your blood pressure at home, tell your doctor. It may also be better to check your blood pressure less often.

Borderline and Mild Hypertension

In diagnosing hypertension, physicians and patients alike prefer a clear diagnosis: Either your blood pressure is above 140/90 and you have hypertension, or it is below and you do not. I wish that diagnosing hypertension were that straightforward.

It would be nice to believe that there are two distinct populations: one with a normal blood pressure and one with hypertension. However, it is illogical to believe that someone with a blood pressure of 141/91 has a disease called hypertension that will lead to a stroke or heart attack and someone with a blood pressure of 139/89 does not. In fact, their risk is essentially the same and is affected more by other factors such as smoking, high cholesterol, diabetes, and family history than by the slight elevation in blood pressure. If a patient has such risk factors, I tend to treat even minimal hypertension. If they don't, the risk of complications from borderline hypertension and the benefit of treating it are much smaller.

BLOOD PRESSURE VARIES constantly in everyone, and can vary considerably from day to day, even from minute to minute. Therefore, it is usually impossible to diagnose hypertension based on one or two or three readings. A single elevated reading often returns to normal on its own, without any treatment.

In a review in 1971, Stevo Julius concluded that half of people with borderline hypertension never develop hypertension. Large studies, such as the Medical Research Council trial in England, reported in the *British Medical Journal* in 1985, and the Australian study, reported in *Lancet* in 1980, show that in a third of people with mild hypertension the blood pressure returns to normal without any treatment. This is why treatment for mild hypertension is not recommended until elevated readings have persisted for three to six months. Unfortunately, this dictum is often ignored, often because of exaggerated concern about the immediate risk of mild blood pressure elevation.

As a specialist in hypertension, I find the toughest decisions to make are whether to prescribe medication for people with the mildest hypertension. The need for treatment is much less clear than in people with more severe hypertension. The commitment to spend thousands of dollars for years or decades of pills is often hard to justify, simply because the blood pressure is a few millimeters above an arbitrary criterion.

Since the complications of mild hypertension take place only after years or decades, there is no harm in deferring medication for a few months and trying nondrug measures first. Lifestyle changes can often help avoid the need for long-term medication, as I will discuss in Chapter 13.

Temporary Hypertension

Why do one out of three people with untreated mild hypertension end up with normal blood pressure reading without any treatment? It may be due partly to the fading of the alerting phenomenon I discussed earlier. I believe it also reflects the temporary nature of blood pressure elevation in many people. The common belief that once hypertensive, always hypertensive, is often incorrect.

In many people, hypertension can be temporary. If your blood pressure is elevated at a time of major upheaval, it may often return to normal on its own, days or weeks later. Sometimes, even if there is no obvious reason for its rise, it can still fall back to normal.

For this reason, if your blood pressure is well controlled on medication, it is often worthwhile to see, under the supervision of a physician, if it will remain normal without medication. If you are basically healthy and have mild hypertension, you will not get into trouble doing this. If your blood pressure goes up, you can resume the medication. If not, you can remain off it, although you should check your blood pressure every few weeks to make sure it does not creep back up over time.

Many patients come to me believing that all of their blood pressure readings are supposed to be normal. This is also not true. Studies using a computerized blood pressure monitor show that almost everyone has some elevated readings during the course of the day, depending on variations in activity or emotion. The diagnosis of hypertension is not made on the basis of a few high readings. It is based on the average blood pressure—on what your blood pressure is most of the time.

The more often you measure your blood pressure, particularly at moments of stress, the more likely you will encounter some high readings. This is often the case when hypertension is suddenly discovered during an emergency room visit for treatment of, for example, a bad laceration. It is important to know what the blood pressure is at other times, and to not diagnose and treat based on an isolated reading at a bad moment. If you check your blood pressure only at moments of stress, it will inevitably lead to overestimation of your usual blood pressure, and possibly to a misdiagnosis of hypertension and unnecessary treatment.

Even if you truly have hypertension and require medication, you may be on more medication than you need. I see many patients with well-controlled hypertension whose medication was increased because of an occasional elevated reading at their doctor's office. Typically they tell me that "the medication stopped working" or "I became immune to the medication," when in fact their blood pressure was still normal most of the time.

It is wrong to misinterpret an occasional elevated reading as treatment failure. Your blood pressure can fluctuate no matter how many pills you take. Antihypertensive medications do not prevent this.

Unless the elevation is extreme or persistent, you should manage it by monitoring your blood pressure, rather than rushing to increase your medication. Sometimes a change in medication is necessary. However, in many instances the blood pressure will return to its usual level without any intervention.

The Physician's Attitude

We have talked about patients' attitudes about their blood pressure. What about physicians' attitudes? How might your physician's attitude affect the measurement of your blood pressure?

▶ One day, Ruth, eighty-six, whose blood pressure had always been normal, was told by her physician that it was 170/90. He warned her that this was dangerously high and prescribed medication. Her son-in-law, a patient of mine, asked me whether I concurred with the decision to treat her blood pressure.

Ruth's life was no different from two years ago when her blood pressure was perfectly normal. There was no reason to believe she had suddenly developed hypertension. I was surprised that the medication had been started after only one elevated reading and suggested that she stop the medication and come in to see me.

In my office, her blood pressure, off medication, was 125/75, which is very normal. I advised her to stay off the medication and have her blood pressure checked in another month.

She saw me a month later. Her physician had obtained another reading of 170/90 and again insisted that she should be on medication. In my office, her blood pressure was 130/75.

Two years later, Ruth remains off medication. Her blood pressure has remained very normal. ◄

Ruth's case demonstrates a phenomenon that I believe frequently occurs in doctors' offices but is not discussed in medical journals. It shows how blood pressure can be elevated when people see one physician but not another.

I see many patients whose blood pressure might be 160/100 when it is checked by other physicians and 120/80 in my office. I see others whose blood pressure is elevated when they see me and normal when they see their gynecologist or other physician. Some patients conclude that the gynecologist doesn't know how to measure blood pressure. I usually conclude that the patient was probably less focused on her blood pressure when the gynecologist checked it and that the gynecologist's measurement probably better reflects her usual blood pressure.

Measurements in the doctor's office are particularly likely to overestimate the blood pressure in elderly people. In a report in 1988, Michael Ruddy found the white coat phenomenon in over 40 percent of elderly people who had elevated readings in the doctor's office. His findings suggest caution in making long-term treatment decisions.

Ruth's case also demonstrates that the attitude of the physician can have an important effect on the readings. When a physician, even a well-meaning one, frightens a patient into believing that she is at imminent risk of having a stroke, that she is a "ticking time bomb," the readings can often be higher than they would otherwise have been. A more appropriate attitude, reflecting the modest increase in risk in people with mild hypertension and the low risk of an imminent event, is less likely to have this effect.

Why do some doctors use scare tactics? Some feel they motivate patients to take their medication. However, they can also lead people to stay away from doctors and medicine.

A physician's attitude can fan the flames of the alerting reaction, causing future readings to be elevated, and confirming the misdiagnosed hypertension and the need for medication. Even the serious facial expression, without a word spoken, unwittingly conveys this fear. That is why checking your blood pressure outside the doctor's office is often a necessity for optimal treatment.

How to Tell if You Truly Have Hypertension

If you have severely elevated blood pressure, or if you have clear evidence of damage caused by hypertension, such as kidney damage, thickening of the heart wall on electrocardiogram or echocardiogram, changes in the small arteries in the eyes, or other signs, it is clear that you need long-term treatment. Otherwise, I would first want to assess the possibility that you have an alerting reaction or temporary hypertension.

If you have mild hypertension, I cannot advise you strongly enough to obtain readings *outside your physician's office* before starting long-term medication. You might be pleasantly surprised to find out that you do not truly have hypertension.

There are many ways to monitor your blood pressure outside your physician's office. The best ways are either to check your own blood pressure at work or at home, or to wear an ambulatory monitor for a day.

You can check your own blood pressure at home by purchasing a monitor at a drugstore or surgical supply store, at a cost in the range of $100. The most accurate ones are the mercury or anaeroid types, but these require listening through a stethoscope for the appearance and disappearance of the Korotkoff sounds. Computerized devices that provide a digital readout are more convenient. These devices are now quite accurate, although you should bring your apparatus to your physician's office to confirm its accuracy.

In general, you can consider your home readings to be normal if they average about 130/85 or lower. Some of your readings will likely be higher, but that should not provoke a rush to treatment.

Many patients ask me when is the best time of day to check their blood pressure. On average, blood pressure is slightly higher in the morning than in the evening, but everyone has their own pattern. It is reasonable to check it at different times.

It can be informative to check your blood pressure when you think it is up, such as when you are upset, to determine if your feeling matches the actual reading. However, if you check it only when you are upset, your readings might not reflect your usual pressure. Therefore, be sure to also check it at random times.

If you get extremely nervous even when you check your blood pressure at home, you should mention this to your doctor. Your readings might not reflect your true blood pressure. I would also suggest that you not check your blood pressure twenty times a day. Once a week, or even less, is enough, unless you have severe hypertension or are changing medications.

Physicians who specialize in treating hypertension can also check your blood pressure with a computerized ambulatory monitor. This type of monitor consists of a cuff that is placed on your arm and is attached to a small control device that automatically inflates the cuff, recording your blood pressure every fifteen to thirty minutes throughout a twenty-four-hour period. The readings obtained provide a good profile of your usual blood pressure throughout the day and night.

BEFORE YOU STRUGGLE to understand why you have hypertension and before you accept the need for lifelong medication, make sure that you truly have hypertension. Even if your doctor is the best doctor in the world, it is usually wise to confirm that you have hypertension with readings outside of the medical office.

The False Promise of Popular Beliefs about Stress and Hypertension

3

> ► Barbara, forty-four, came to see me after another doctor had told her that her blood pressure was high. There were many reasons for her to have hypertension. In addition to a strong family history of hypertension, Barbara, at five foot three, weighed 220 pounds and emotionally was a wreck. Her husband had left her for another woman four years ago, and she was still very agitated, angry, and depressed. At times she felt suicidal. She was at a maximum of emotional distress.
>
> Her blood pressure was 114/80, very normal. ◄

WHEN I SEE patients like Barbara, I just cannot believe that the emotions we feel are a major cause of hypertension. I have seen this pattern again and again. Patients tell me they are completely "stressed out" and yet their blood pressure has hardly risen from its usual level. In this chapter I shall describe how my clinical experience and the bulk of reported research converge to the same conclusion: The mind–body link of hypertension cannot be found if we limit our search to the emotional distress people feel.

Stress and Blood Pressure: Fluctuation Versus Hypertension

Considerable research about mental stress and hypertension focuses on the increase in blood pressure following stress administered in a laboratory. We call this *blood pressure reactivity*. The beauty of such experiments is that the researcher can administer the identical stress to every subject in a study, and then easily measure and compare the blood pressure responses. In this way, the study of stress can be converted to numbers, to scientific data. Thousands of such studies tell us unequivocally that mental stress briefly raises blood pressure. They also tell us that the blood pressure falls back down very quickly.

Stresses such as mental arithmetic and video games are widely used to test blood pressure reactivity in the laboratory. They raise blood pressure about 10 to 20 millimeters, even in people who don't have hypertension. Many investigators have sought to show that the magnitude of this blood pressure response identifies people who are prone to hypertension. Reviews of this research indicate that it does not.

Guido Grassi, in a recent review of studies of blood pressure reactivity published in the *Journal of Hypertension* in 1996, reached several disturbing conclusions about this large body of research. He noted, for example, that a person can have a large blood pressure response to one stressor and a minimal one to another, or a variable response to the very same stressor. He also concluded that the magnitude of the blood pressure response to laboratory stress bears little relationship to the magnitude of the response to real-life stress. Gianfranco Parati showed that a person's blood pressure reactivity in the laboratory bears little relationship to his blood pressure or its variability throughout the day. Reviews by David Krantz in 1984, Thomas Pickering in 1990, Kathy Light in 1981, and others similarly conclude that measuring blood pressure reactivity in the laboratory does not predict whether hypertension will develop.

Studies also show that in real life as well the distress we feel temporarily elevates our blood pressure. Gary James reported in 1986 that, throughout the day, blood pressure rises when people are angry or sad, and falls when they are happy.

Studies show that feeling anxious or angry, or expressing our emotions, briefly raises blood pressure but doesn't lead to hypertension. If anything, the reviews of Randall Jorgensen in 1996 and Jerry Suls in 1995 reveal that people who express their anger tend to have a lower rather than higher blood pressure than others. The classic story, reported by Stewart Wolf in 1948, is of a man whose blood pressure fell from 165/100 to 125/85 after beating up his brother-in-law!

Thousands of studies have sought to prove that people who tend to feel angry or tense or depressed eventually develop hypertension. Their results have been extremely inconsistent and support all points of view on the subject. Many reviews note this inconsistency (some examples are reviews by Chris Cottier, 1987; Randall Jorgensen, 1996; Jerry Suls, 1995; Eric Cottington, 1985; and Mary Monk, 1980). Like the emperor's clothes, the supposed link between the emotions we feel and hypertension is less apparent than we think.

Some have suggested that brief increases in blood pressure, repeated many times over years, eventually lead to structural changes in blood vessels and permanent elevation of blood pressure. Here as well, review after review concedes that the evidence is weak (some examples are reviews by Alan Weder, 1985, and Herb Weiner, 1987).

A logical argument against this belief can also be gleaned from what happens to blood pressure during physical labor. During the physical stress of manual labor, blood pressure increases substantially and repeatedly throughout the day, often to levels much higher than during emotional stress. Yet people who have done physical labor for decades are no more prone to develop hypertension than anyone else. If mild blood pressure elevation from repeated emotional stress could lead to hypertension, these frequent and often greater elevations would also be expected to lead to hypertension, and they don't.

Many studies look at the effects of job stress. Certainly the emotional and physical frenzy of work will raise blood pressure somewhat during the workday. We cannot expect our blood pressure to be the same as if we were home, sitting and reading a book. However, several studies, such as one reported by Thalina

Lindquist in the journal *Hypertension* in 1997, have failed to show that this mild elevation, which occurs even in people who don't have hypertension, results in hypertension. Other studies, such as one by Marilyn Winkleby in 1988, also show that people with hypertension are no more distressed by work than anyone else. Thus, I believe that studies of job stress will not solve a big piece of the hypertension mystery.

Many patients ask me whether exercise, during which our blood pressure increases substantially, could be harmful. Studies show that regular aerobic exercise can help keep blood pressure down (see G. Kelley, 1994, and R. Fagard, 1995). Even a regimen of weight lifting might lead to lower blood pressure (see R. L. Wiley, 1992). The only time I hesitate to recommend exercise, particularly vigorous exercise, is in people who have severe hypertension, until it has been lowered somewhat.

Moving from studies to real life, I find the same thing: Most people who have hypertension, even severe hypertension, don't complain of feeling more emotional distress than anyone else. The person who has severe hypertension and complains of severe emotional distress is the exception, not the rule.

We Are Wired to Handle Stress

My own experience with thousands of patients supports these conclusions. My patients' blood pressure usually does not seem closely related to how tense they tell me they are feeling, or to how much stress they are under. I see examples of this again and again.

> ► Doug, a slim forty-three-year-old businessman, had a minimally elevated blood pressure of 130/90 at his first visit to me. Since his blood pressure had always been normal, he was not very concerned about it.
>
> He came to see me two months later while under severe job-related stress. He had been sleeping poorly and was also worried about his blood pressure. He was certain it would be elevated. To his amazement it was 115/75. ◄

Almost daily, patients will tell me they are having a terribly stressful week or month and expect their blood pressure to be higher than usual. Occasionally it is, but usually it is not. Every day patients tell me their blood pressure will be high because they had to combat New York City traffic driving to my office. It never is. It was probably higher while they were sitting in traffic and cursing, but probably by the time they parked their car it was back down.

The opposite is also true. Patients who tell me they have had a wonderful week or month, have had no stress, and expect their blood pressure to be down usually have the same readings as before.

After seeing this pattern day in and day out, I cannot believe that routine day-to-day stress has much to do with the development of essential hypertension. The emotions we feel do have brief effects but not long-lasting ones. Despite the expectations of most of the researchers doing this work, we can only conclude that these emotions do not provide an explanation for essential hypertension. Beverly's story is a compelling example.

▶ Beverly, a slim sixty-year-old brunette, was a happily married mother of two grown children. She lived in an affluent community surrounded by good friends. She had borderline hypertension, with readings in my office of 140–150/70–80 over a two-year period. Since she had no other cardiovascular risk factors, such as high cholesterol or smoking, and since her readings were slightly lower when measured at home, I had not prescribed medication.

At a routine visit, she informed me that her daughter had been found to have an advanced stage of malignant melanoma, a fatal type of skin cancer. She was trying to be optimistic but was fully aware of the prognosis. She cried in my office, describing how her life could never be the same. Her blood pressure, surprising both of us, was unchanged.

During the next year, Beverly's life was dominated by her daughter's illness. She read all she could about melanoma and sought the best doctors and the most promising experimental treatments. She became more knowledgeable about melanoma than most doctors. She also became her daughter's main caretaker through course after course of chemotherapy. However, she knew that no matter what she did and how much she hoped, her daughter was likely to die.

I have no idea how people cope with a stress of this magnitude and did not know what to say to her. I hoped her daughter would recover but never reassured Beverly that she would. I knew I couldn't. Trying to paint a rosy picture to bypass her discomfort would offer false reassurance. Since I did not want to offer trite advice, I tended to listen sympathetically more than talk.

I came to admire Beverly's ability to feel the distress and yet function, and to dedicate her time with her daughter to her daughter's needs rather than to her own. Beverly seemed to have the emotional strength to feel her distress and not fall apart. I said this to her and she seemed strengthened by my awareness of her strength. We shared a sense of connectedness.

After a year, her daughter died. During that year Beverly's blood pressure was not one millimeter higher than it was before. She will feel the pain of her loss until the day she dies, but she has recovered from the grief, and is active and radiant. ◄

I don't care how much the stress of mental arithmetic raises blood pressure in a research laboratory. Two minutes of mental arithmetic would likely have raised Beverly's blood pressure 10 or 20 millimeters. Yet the year-long stress of her daughter's fatal illness did not. This paradox demonstrates how little the blood pressure response to brief distress has to do with the response to prolonged distress. Although our blood pressure rises and falls continuously in response to day-to-day stress, this phenomenon has little to do with the tendency to develop hypertension.

Beverly faced a greater stress and experienced greater distress than any laboratory can produce, and did so for a full year. After monitoring her blood pressure throughout that year and seeing reactions in other severely distressed patients with similarly minimal increases in blood pressure, I come again and again to the same conclusion: The emotions we feel cannot be a major determinant of hypertension.

It is our destiny to encounter stress throughout our lives, and I believe we are wired to handle it. Our autonomic nervous system, which consists of the nerves that connect our brain to our cardiovascular system and which regulates our blood pressure, is wired to handle what we feel without permanently distorting our blood pressure.

Do Relaxation Techniques Help?

The belief that the distressing emotions we feel cause hypertension led naturally to the belief that reducing or controlling these emotions would help treat it. Herbert Benson showed that transcendental meditation can lower blood pressure, as he described in 1977 in his book *The Relaxation Response*. Biofeedback, relaxation techniques, and stress reduction techniques can similarly lower blood pressure.

The problem with most of these methods is that their effects are short-lived. Just as the emotions we feel briefly raise our blood pressure, these techniques briefly lower it. Removing ourselves from active physical and emotional engagement, even without relaxation techniques, will also lower blood pressure. If you can do biofeedback or relaxation techniques all day, it will lower your blood pressure all day. Obviously this is not feasible.

The more important question is whether these techniques have a persisting effect on blood pressure. Many uncontrolled studies suggest that they do. However, better controlled studies conclude that they don't (for example, see Trials of Hypertension Prevention, 1992; S. N. Hunyor, 1996). A major review by David Eisenberg, published in the *Annals of Internal Medicine* in 1993, found that, on average, relaxation techniques lowered systolic blood pressure by only 2 millimeters and diastolic pressure by 1 millimeter.

Blood pressure readings in a physician's office or clinic often settle down on their own, no matter how effective or ineffective the intervention being tested. For this reason, studies must compare the response to any intervention with changes seen in an untreated control group. In addition, since home readings are less subject to a placebo effect, it is important that studies also assess the effect of an intervention on blood pressure measured outside the clinic. Recent studies find that the effect of relaxation techniques is not evident in blood pressure monitored throughout the day (see studies reported by R. G. Jacob, 1992; G. A. Montfrans, 1990; and D. W. Johnston, 1993). An encouraging study by Charles Alexander reported in 1996 found a 10 millimeter fall in home systolic blood pressure with transcendental meditation. I await other studies to confirm or refute this result.

Reviewing the studies, the 1993 and 1997 reports of the Joint National Committee on the Detection, Evaluation and Treatment of High Blood Pressure, comprising the views of leading hypertension experts in the United States, did not recommend these techniques. They concluded: "The available literature does not support the use of relaxation therapies for definitive therapy or prevention of hypertension."

My experience with patients is very consistent with the results of controlled studies. I see many patients whose blood pressure settles down on its own. I have seen few who have had sustained improvement through relaxation techniques. Relaxation techniques can be very helpful in reducing emotional distress but generally should not be relied on to control hypertension.

Solving the Mind–Body Mystery

What Are Hidden Emotions?

4

I HAVE LEARNED from my patients that what I call "hidden" emotions have much more to do with hypertension than do the emotions we feel. These are the emotions that we do not feel and often are not aware that we harbor within us. Since we are not distressed by them, it would never occur to us that they are affecting us physically. At first it was hard to believe. However, the more experience I have gathered, the more frequently I have been able to see this link between hidden emotions and hypertension, and the path it offers to healing.

The evidence for the role of hidden emotions did not come from textbooks. Nor can hidden emotions be easily measured in the laboratory. Ironically, uncovering the role of hidden emotions did not require high technology. It required neither electricity nor computers nor a microscope. It required simply listening to people and their stories, and listening to what they were saying and what they were not saying. Their stories opened the door to making sense of their hypertension.

The Calm Masquerade

▶ I was treating Bill, a stocky man of fifty-five, for both mild hypertension and diabetes. He was five-nine and weighed 230 pounds. On medication, his blood pressure was consistently normal, never higher than 130/85. He felt well but regularly complained about job stress.

In 1992 Bill began to experience chest discomfort and I admitted him to the hospital for cardiac catheterization to assess his coronary arteries. It was scheduled to be done two days later.

During those two days he felt perfectly well, but his blood pressure hovered at 170/110 much of the time, a striking 40/25 millimeters above his usual. This was unusual because bed rest in a hospital usually lowers blood pressure.

The logical explanation was that Bill was anxious about the upcoming procedure. However, he insisted he was not. I mentioned that his blood pressure elevation suggested anxiety, and reassured him that some degree of anxiety was natural and normal. He again insisted he was not worried at all, that he felt fine.

The catheterization was performed without complication and revealed no coronary artery disease. I visited Bill afterward, while he was lying on a stretcher with a sandbag compressing the puncture site in his groin. He told me he was relieved that he would not need surgery. Then his face contorted, like the face of a child when taken over by a loud cry. He began to cry, telling me how scared he had been during the catheterization. He quickly felt better. His blood pressure is once again normal. ◄

Bill's blood pressure had been markedly elevated for two days, for no apparent reason. If he had acknowledged being anxious during those two days, any physician would have readily attributed the blood pressure elevation to anxiety.

Even though Bill claimed he did not feel anxious prior to the catheterization, I believe anxiety, even though hidden from his awareness, was the cause of his blood pressure elevation. There was no other explanation for it. This case showed me that people can be harboring considerable anxiety even if they don't *feel* anxious, and that this anxiety, even if not felt, can have a considerable effect on blood pressure.

Two years later, Bill still insisted he had not been frightened during those two days. His blood pressure had revealed otherwise.

Another case similarly demonstrates that what is completely hidden can affect our blood pressure.

▸ Celia was a fifty-year-old business school student determined to get her MBA. She described herself as "high-strung." She had borderline hypertension. Her blood pressure, monitored automatically every fifteen minutes for a twenty-four-hour period, averaged 140/88, slightly above normal. I was considering starting her on medication.

After an absence of several months, she returned to my office and described having suffered the night before, "out of the blue," a thirty-minute episode of sudden, severe blood pressure elevation, reaching 200/110, accompanied by a headache and shortness of breath. She had then rushed to an emergency room near her home and received medication that quickly lowered her blood pressure.

Celia had never had such a high reading and felt there was no apparent reason for it. She told me she had been relaxed at the time it occurred and felt the episode was not related to stress.

Celia related to me that she had been discharged from the hospital only a week earlier following surgery for a recently discovered colon cancer. She stated, however, that she was not anxious about the cancer and that she was certain the attack was not caused by anxiety. Interestingly, I recalled from her family history that her mother had died of colon cancer at age fifty! ◂

Cancer is obviously a major stress, particularly in someone whose mother died of the same cancer at the same age. Yet Celia insisted she was not worried about it and appeared quite unconcerned. She was not telling me that she had gone through a period of upset and had gradually calmed down. She was not telling me that she was worried but trying to avoid her feelings. She was telling me that she had no troubling feelings. She *knew* she had this cancer but was not upset about it.

I noted three features in Celia's case and subsequently in many others: a severe stress, the conspicuous absence of the emotional distress that would have been expected, and the conspicuous and otherwise unexplained elevation of blood pressure. Like Bill, if

Celia had acknowledged being frightened, any physician would have attributed the blood pressure spike to the emotion. Her case also suggested that emotions can elevate blood pressure even when we don't feel them, that our body reacts to our emotions even when, or perhaps especially when, we are unaware of them. Celia's blood pressure was telling me more about her emotional state than her words.

BILL AND CELIA each had a conspicuous source of severe stress. Nothing in their manner told me of the emotional distress hidden within. The only clue lay in the stressful situations confronting them.

In many other people, the source of hidden distress fueling longer-lasting blood pressure elevation is not as readily apparent. It could be an abusive marriage that a woman accepts as okay, or any other stress that people don't even mention to me because, remarkably, they do not feel upset. The absence of an obvious source for hidden anxiety is not proof that there is no such source.

I began to look differently at many other cases. I realized that patients' testimony that they are not feeling distress does not necessarily mean that emotions are not causing their hypertension. Such distress, even if severe, could be concealed from both the patient and from me. Ironically, such patients, like Celia, are certain that stress is not playing a role in their hypertension.

The role of hidden emotions is not easy to discern. People cannot tell their physicians about them, and troubling emotions usually are not mentioned even during careful discussion. Their effect on blood pressure is also obscured by the temporary but more immediate and obvious effects of the emotions we do feel, and by many other factors including obesity, alcohol intake, and genetics.

Physicians, patients, and researchers are not accustomed to approaching the mystery of hypertension this way. There is a natural tendency to focus on what patients say they feel. People in scientific circles resist considering the role of hidden emotions. Medical researchers tend to reject their relevance because they cannot see or measure them. The prevailing attitude is that anything that cannot be quantitated cannot be important.

Most physicians and patients accept hypertension as a mystery without even considering that our unconscious mind can affect our health even more than our conscious mind does. As Carl Jung stated in *The Undiscovered Self*, "The unconscious has been ignored altogether . . . not the result of carelessness or the lack of knowledge, but of downright resistance to the mere possibility that there could be a second psychic authority besides the ego. It seems a positive menace to the ego that its monarchy could be doubted."

This attitude still stands true today and is a formidable barrier to more fully understanding the mind–body connection of health and illness.

Our Defenses Against Feeling Our Emotions

We face many unwanted emotions in life. We choose to feel some and to purposely divert our attention from others. Still others we divert from our awareness without any conscious effort, without even knowing we are doing so. Our most powerful emotions are in this category, yet we rarely consider their effect on us and on our health.

We can all acknowledge that there are times when we intentionally divert our attention from emotions we don't want to feel. We know we harbor these emotions inside and that we are avoiding them. For example, if we are feeling sad because of an ended romance, we know we can choose to immerse ourselves in work to avoid the emotional pain.

However, we are much less able and willing to acknowledge that there are times when we block out emotions without even knowing it. We don't know we are avoiding these emotions and hiding them inside. Like Bill and Celia, we would swear up and down that we don't feel them. It is the difference between saying "I prefer not to think about such and such" and saying "No, I don't have those feelings."

Sometimes when we are experiencing extremely painful emotions we are at first aware of our effort to avoid them. Over time we are able to do so more automatically without any awareness or conscious effort. In this way we block out emotions that we may have felt at one time, thinking we have put them completely behind us.

The balance between feeling and avoiding deeply painful emotions is important in how someone handles, for example, the grief of the sudden and tragic loss of a loved one. If the grief descended all at once in its entirety, it might be unbearable and could leave us unable to function. If we instead protect ourselves by blocking out the worst of the pain and letting it in as we are ready, we can continue to function even as we grieve and heal from our loss. Some might never let themselves feel those emotions, and, without realizing it, conceal them within, ultimately becoming unaware of them. They put the trauma behind them but do not heal.

This book is mostly about people who, like Bill and Celia, don't know they are concealing painful emotions and insist that they feel fine. It is usually not hard to recognize that a person has blocked emotions related to very painful events, past or current. Such a person does not get teary talking about the event, no matter how horrible it was. He will insist that the past is the past and that he put the past behind him. He will insist that events from years or decades ago, no matter how traumatic, could not be affecting him today. It is this adamant insistence that there are no lingering emotions or effects that gives the game away.

As I will discuss, I first observed this link between hypertension and hidden emotions where it was easiest to discern: in people with severe hypertension or a history of severe emotional trauma. I later observed it in people with a history of less obvious emotional trauma and with less severe hypertension. Finally, I came to recognize it in people who, even without a history of overt emotional trauma, tend in general to block out many of the distressful emotions of day-to-day life.

I shall begin with the dramatic cases that first opened my eyes to this link.

The Emotional Trauma Locked Inside Us

5

IF THE EMOTIONAL DISTRESS we feel were the cause of hypertension, I would have expected people with the most severe hypertension to feel the most distressed. However, I have not found this to be the case at all. Most people with severe hypertension do not seem to feel more emotionally distressed, or to be under more stress, than anyone else. The emotions they tell me about rarely make sense of their hypertension. The mind–body link is evident only if we stop to consider what is hidden inside.

Trauma Locked Away Inside Us

▶ Leonard, sixty, had severe and uncontrollable hypertension for over twenty years. Even on a combination of four medications, his blood pressure was extremely high: 200/100. Extensive and repeated diagnostic tests had not found a cause.

There was little stress in his life. He was happily married and had three grown children, all of whom were well. He was semi-retired and financially comfortable.

Since current stress could not make sense of his severe hypertension, I inquired about his past, looking for something far outside the norm, something extremely jarring. It made sense to look back more than twenty years, before the onset of his hypertension. He described how his first house burned down shortly after he had returned from military duty. Then he mentioned the sudden accidental death of his first child at the age of nine, twenty-four years ago, after being accidentally hit in the head by a baseball bat.

I asked Leonard about his grief. He replied that he had not grieved, other than crying for a few seconds. He had "put it behind him." He was not saying he had grieved and then moved on. He was saying he had not grieved.

The time frame of this event fit precisely the time frame of his hypertension. The absence of conscious distress, of sharing that distress with anyone, had prevented discharge of that emotion. I had to conclude that the grief was still concealed within him.

I commented to Leonard that I was wondering if his unexplained severe hypertension might be related to these emotions. It seemed logical that exploring these emotions and discharging some of them might be helpful in gaining control of his hypertension. Since this would be very painful, I left the decision to Leonard.

At the next visit Leonard told me that he wanted to leave it alone. I complied with his wishes. I revised his medications and his blood pressure is better, though still above normal. He remains on four medications. ◄

I saw in Leonard, and in other patients, the same coincidence of severe emotional trauma, conspicuous absence of the expected emotional reaction, and development of severe and otherwise unexplained hypertension. I noted the stark contrast in outcome between Leonard and Beverly, whose story I described in Chapter 3. Both had endured the loss of a child. Beverly suffered severe distress and grief, and her blood pressure did not budge. Leonard felt little or no grief and his blood pressure has been severely elevated ever since.

In this case and, subsequently, in many others, where inquiry into current stress could not make sense of severe hypertension, hidden emotions related to previously encountered traumatic life events offered a cogent explanation. A man with both asthma and hypertension for eight years had no current stress to explain them. However, he claimed he emerged emotionally unscathed eight years ago from the simultaneous deaths of both his wife and his mother, and the bankruptcy of his business. Another man with severe hypertension recalls that his mother died suddenly of pneumonia when he was twelve and he was then shipped off to Indiana to live with an aunt. He learned to live his life without letting things bother him, the same way he did not let his mother's death bother him.

Many of the patients I see who have severe hypertension and who have suffered severe emotional trauma in the past insist, almost verbatim, that they have "put it behind" them. They rarely, if ever, suspect that traumatic events from the past could have anything to do with their hypertension, no matter what they have been through.

This response differs glaringly from that of people who have not blocked the emotional reaction in its entirety. In them, even though ultimately they did recover emotionally, mention of the event will provoke a teariness or a response such as "You never completely get over it."

My experience suggested to me that in survivors of emotional trauma there was a reciprocal relationship between emotional distress and hypertension. The more easily they could acknowledge a lingering emotional impact, even a small one, the less likely they were to have developed hypertension, and vice versa.

The patient with the most uncontrollable hypertension I have ever encountered illustrates this further.

▸ Juan's blood pressure was checked for the first time when he was forty-five. It was very high and, since then, he had been prescribed many complicated combinations of medication, all of which had failed to lower it. He was hospitalized repeatedly and had to stop working. Despite all efforts, his hypertension remained uncontrollable, often with readings of 250/150 no matter what medication he took.

Extensive testing had failed to find a cause. His mother and two sisters had hypertension, but genetics could not explain its unusual severity.

Juan was sixty when I met him. He was five foot five and chunky, perhaps 180 pounds. He acknowledged that he had always been nervous, that occasionally his hands would shake uncontrollably.

He also acknowledged being sad. He felt it was just his personality. He said he was always attracted to the clown with the sad face. He could look at that clown's face and cry, but he did not know why.

There was no great stress in his life other than his hypertension. He had been happily married for forty years and his family felt close to him. He loved them very much. For fifteen years he had been a born-again Christian. He struck me as a man of tremendous faith and goodness.

Although his current situation revealed no major source of stress, his early life did. His childhood in the Dominican Republic had not been a happy one. He was the youngest of five children. His father had died when he was one, and his mother subsequently remarried. She had not been warm to him, never hugging or kissing him. He clearly was not her favorite.

His family was poor. Often suffering from hunger, he was at times too weak to get out of his chair.

The only one who paid any attention to Juan was his older brother, Tony. Juan said he had considered Tony his "favorite" brother, until Tony started doing some terrible things. Juan had not talked about it for most of his life but told me that he had briefly mentioned it to a minister two years ago and felt relieved. He felt he had gotten it all out.

Juan then told me the story. Tony would frequently accompany Juan to the shower and abuse him there. Sexually. Painfully. Juan often bled afterward. Tony accompanied him to school and would abuse him in the bushes. A teacher once asked him why he was bleeding. In front of his brother Juan said he had fallen. The teacher probably knew he was lying but thought he had been fooling around.

He told his mother, but she said she didn't believe him. If he cried about anything, he was told not to cry.

The abuse stopped when Tony entered the military and was killed, when Juan was eleven. Juan told me that the day he was told of his brother's death he feigned grief but was happy inside. Juan confessed that he still felt he was partly responsible for the abuse, although the minister he had spoken with had told him it was not his fault.

Juan went on to describe further the unfairness of his childhood. The starvation he had mentioned had an unusual twist: While Juan's dinner was water and a slice of bread with or without sugar, the others ate. Not well, but they ate. Juan worked five hours a day after school. He cleaned their neighbor's house. The others did not.

His mother, years later at her deathbed, asked for his forgiveness. Juan forgave. Everyone asked him why his mother was asking for forgiveness. It was just a family thing, he told them, quickly dropping it.

In talking to me, Juan felt he was pouring out his heart. He laid out the facts in great detail, but did so without showing any deep feeling, without shedding a tear.

He told me he feared that if he started crying he would never stop. Though he did not feel these emotions, he suspected they were not deeply buried. He was afraid of them. The nine-year-old child in his heart was in severe and eternal torment, and to this day no one was willing to hear his screams of pain or fury, not even the adult Juan. The battle inside to keep those emotions out of awareness was becoming more and more costly. I suspect this is why his hypertension was so severe.

Juan chose not to talk further and declined the option of psychotherapy. I had hoped he would eventually choose to engage some of the emotions, but the decision to engage the horror of his past had to be his, not mine.

Juan's hypertension remained severe and uncontrollable. He died from its complications two years later. ◄

Juan's trauma had been severe. He was not completely isolated from his emotions, but the sadness he felt did not scratch the surface of his boyhood torment, and he did not feel his hidden rage at all. He was struggling to maintain the barrier he had erected as a child to protect him from feeling the brunt of those emotions. He had strengths—his faith in God, his family. He was not alone. However, his trauma had been severe and prolonged in the delicate years of childhood.

I could have looked at every aspect of stress in Juan's current life and would not have come up with an explanation for his unusually severe hypertension. Only in looking at the horrible trauma from childhood—trauma that matched the severity of his hypertension and that he thought he had put behind him decades ago—was a possible explanation evident.

Juan's warmth masked his inner agony. I was saddened that a man of his apparent faith could not heal from the past. In talking with the minister and with me, he had briefly talked about his past but had not scratched the surface of the emotion hidden inside.

Perhaps there is a limit to what we can permit into awareness. Perhaps for Juan, at sixty, it was too late. I hoped that in younger patients, or patients with less severe trauma, that it was not too late.

Breaking Through

Many people, with or without hypertension, can claim a past history that includes emotional trauma. Thus, I do not attribute hypertension to past events simply because someone recalls such an event. In my experience, an important clue that suggests that a previous traumatic event is not just coincidental is when a person insists it had absolutely no lingering emotional impact. This indicates that the emotional impact has been blocked from conscious awareness.

I naturally wondered if the blood pressure would fall if a patient became aware of some of those emotions. However, awareness usually does not come easily or quickly, even in the office of a psychoanalyst. This is why we will never be able to easily study the effect of gaining awareness of blocked emotions in a laboratory. It would also be difficult to attribute a sizable fall in blood pressure to a months-long or years-long process of gaining awareness since antihypertensive medications used in the interim would complicate interpretation of any changes.

Whereas it would be difficult to produce evidence in a laboratory, I believe we can find it in clinical observations. I doubt if I will encounter many cases in which the relationship between hidden emotions and hypertension is as clearly demonstrated as in a patient of mine whose case I reported in *Psychosomatic Medicine* in 1995.

▸ Martha was a forty-nine-year-old woman of average height and weight, who saw me for the first time in 1987. She had severe hypertension and had been hospitalized three times because of it. She had already suffered a stroke, and was lucky that her speech and strength had returned quickly to normal. Nevertheless, she knew she was at high risk of further complications.

Her mother had died of complications of hypertension at age forty-three. Her father had died a few years ago, in his seventies. All of her sisters had hypertension, suggesting that her hypertension was at least partly genetic in origin. However, genetics could not explain its severity.

Martha was taking five antihypertensive medications and there was little left to offer her. Occasionally, her blood pressure was normal, but usually it was not. Often it was extremely elevated, remaining above 170/120 for months at a time, despite all the medication. If she stopped her pills, her blood pressure quickly climbed higher. Intensive diagnostic evaluations had not found a cause.

Martha and I shared many ups and downs in her treatment over the next six years. Whenever her blood pressure came under control and we were about to congratulate ourselves, back up it would go. At first I thought she had not been taking the medication. Occasionally she had not, but even when she took her pills faithfully, her blood pressure could remain extremely high.

Martha had a steady boyfriend. Between their two incomes they were managing, and her life was on a relatively even keel. She had mastered computer skills and had advanced from her entry-level secretarial job. However, because of headaches from her blood pressure and side effects from medication, she was often absent from work. She was worried about her job. Her supervisor, although supportive, could no longer accept her numerous absences.

Toward the end of 1992, her blood pressure had crept up at monthly visits, again reaching 170/120. Her blood pressure at home was similarly elevated, indicating that this was not just white coat hypertension.

One day, upon entering my office, she seemed agitated.

"The extra pill you prescribed last visit is giving me nightmares," Martha told me.

Since I had not prescribed any new medications, I thought it unlikely that the nightmares were related to the pills. I asked, "How long have you been getting the nightmares?"

"The past few weeks."

"Are they different nightmares or does the same nightmare keep recurring?"

"It's the same one. I'm afraid to go to sleep. I sit in the chair in the living room all night. I haven't slept well in weeks."

"What's the nightmare?"

"A man is coming after me. I feel him coming up behind me. Just when I feel him touching my back, I wake up screaming. I'm afraid to go to sleep."

I paused, then asked her, "What man attacked you in the past?"

She hesitated, clearly upset. "I didn't remember this until a month or two ago. I was raped. I can't believe I never remembered it before."

"How old were you?"

"Fourteen."

"And what happened?"

"He was big. He jumped on me and I couldn't move. He hurt me. He hurt me."

"Did you know him?"

"Yes. My uncle."

"Did you tell anyone?"

"My father. He was the only one I could always depend on. He told me he would take care of it. He went to the police, but nothing happened. They told him they didn't want to make a big family thing out of it. We should keep it to ourselves."

"Did anything happen after that?"

"No. No one said anything about it. My aunt and uncle separated, and I haven't seen him in years. If I ever see him, I'll kill him."

"Do you remember anything else? Did you see a doctor?"

"I know I was in the hospital sometime around then. I guess it was shortly after that."

"What was the problem?"

"I had an infection in my womb."

"How long were you in the hospital?"

"They kept me for two weeks. They were giving me antibiotics."

"Do you think the nightmares might be connected to regaining memory of the rape? They seem to have begun around the same time."

"Maybe. I didn't think about that."

I asked her what might have triggered her recollection of the rape. She described how the memory arose while glancing at her cousin, her uncle's child. She had suddenly noticed her uncle's features in the child's maturing face.

We talked a little longer, after which I checked her blood pressure. It was 220/150. She felt okay except for a mild headache. She was accustomed to a high blood pressure level and was able to tolerate this extra elevation.

Her blood pressure was the same a half hour later. I wanted to admit her to the hospital. She wanted to go home. After additional medication, her pressure fell to 150/110, still elevated, but much better. I also called in a social worker who counsels rape victims. Although the event had occurred thirty years earlier, the memory of it and the emotions related to it were new. Martha had essentially been in a state of psychic numbing, with the emotions related to the rape blocked from awareness, protecting her from the distress that probably would have overwhelmed a fourteen-year-old.

She kept on repeating: "I can't believe I told you. I never told anyone."

The rape intervention counselor talked privately with her and encouraged her to come back for follow-up sessions. She agreed. Her blood pressure when she left to go home was back up to 170/120. She promised to return in the morning.

The next morning she felt better. She had had her first good night's sleep in weeks. She had slept so well that she was late for her appointment. Also, for the first time in weeks, she had had no nightmares. I checked her blood pressure. It was 115/85!

Martha's blood pressure, previously impossible to control, remained normal, even after I stopped three of her five medications. The nightmares never returned. She saw the rape counselor regularly for several months, dealing with the issue of her rape and other issues of victimization and assertiveness. She moved out of state eighteen months later, her blood pressure still consistently normal. ◄

Since our blood pressure can rise or fall quite a bit on its own, we have to consider any single case history very cautiously. In Martha's case, however, the rapid, substantial and sustained fall in blood pressure came after years of uncontrollable hypertension, as shown in Figure 5.1. Martha's hypertension, previously uncontrollable on five medications, was now easily controlled on two medications. The dramatic improvement coincided with the emotional disclosure and with cessation of the nightmares, arguing strongly that hidden emotions related to the long-forgotten rape had a lot to do with her hypertension. The swiftness of the fall in Martha's blood pressure after she confided her story was surprising to us both and is an extremely important observation that I shall return to later.

Martha is still amazed that she told me her story. She had always believed that sharing problems is a sign of weakness, that keeping them to yourself is strength.

LIKE MANY of the other severely hypertensive patients I have seen, Martha had dealt with overwhelming trauma by blocking out the related emotions, and, in this case, the memory as well, and mov-

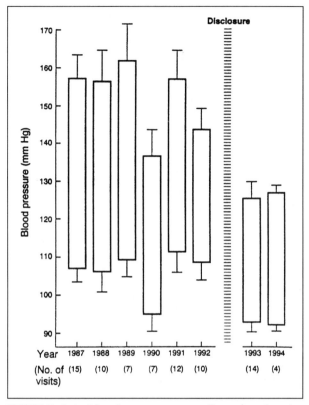

FIGURE 5.1. Blood pressure recordings for the six-year period before, and the eighteen-month period after, disclosure of a decades-old rape. For each year, the upper margin of the bar represents the average systolic blood pressure recorded during that year. The lower margin represents the diastolic pressure. (Reprinted from Mann SJ and Delon M, *Psychosomatic Medicine*, Vol. 57, page 503, 1995.)

ing on. And, since she didn't feel the emotional distress, she had no motivation to look back at that trauma.

Many individuals with severe hypertension don't know that the past revisits them every day, whether they feel it or not. Many don't know that acknowledging the past and the emotions related to it might help their hypertension and perhaps many other aspects of their health.

Martha was unaware of her painful emotions and her fear of feeling them. She would never have guessed that she had the strength now to face them. Her nightmares were the clue that those emotions were coming closer to the surface. Continuing to fight that awareness, like Juan did, would have become a more and more costly battle.

As I will discuss in Chapters 8 and 11, emotions from past events sometimes are truly too overwhelming to be uncovered and should be left alone. However, as you will see from case after case, many of us have more strength than we realize and can now face that which we could not face earlier in our lives. This strength is the key to healing.

Usual Stress Versus Overwhelming Stress

Unless we live in a cocoon, we will certainly encounter stress. The amount of emotional distress it causes us depends both on how much stress we encounter and on how we handle it. Some of us feel extremely distressed when facing minor stress; others thrive in the face of considerable stress.

Most of the stress we encounter is the normal day-to-day stress of living. In the big scheme of things, the traffic jam, the outrageous price we were just charged, and the beautiful weekend we had to spend on the job are not major stresses. We might hate them, but we deal with them and move on. Job stress, arguments with a spouse, aggravation from children, and financial worries are often extremely distressing. We may occasionally feel overwhelmed by them, but, in general, we are "wired" to deal with these as well.

My observations suggest that how we handle these typical stresses of life affects how we feel more than it affects our blood pressure. If we have to deal with a lot of stress, or if we don't cope well with it, we feel distressed, anxious, upset, and tired. Our blood pressure can sometimes increase a bit, but the long-term effect, if any, is small.

Truly overwhelming stress, in contrast, is the type of stress that we are not wired to handle consciously. It can be the stress of severe emotional trauma during childhood or adulthood that attacks us to the core of our emotional stability. Or it might be a lesser stress, if we cope poorly with stress or if a particular stress carries a unique significance.

We are also wired to handle this stress, but in a different way. When we need to, we are wired to block out emotions to avoid being overwhelmed.

When we cannot tolerate feeling the full force of intense emotions, our ability to not feel them protects us. However, it leaves a debt of unfelt, unconsoled emotional pain—a debt with the potential to affect us for the rest of our lives.

The effect might go unnoticed, woven silently in our mood and relationships. It might manifest itself as emotional symptoms such as anxiety or panic disorders, depression, nightmares, or post-traumatic stress disorder. My experience tells me that it can also manifest itself as physical disorders such as hypertension or other unexplained medical conditions. If we pay attention to these disorders as clues of hidden emotions locked inside us, a path to healing is available. If we do not, we may require all sorts of life-long treatments.

These emotions are hard to acknowledge. It makes no sense to most of us that emotions we put behind us long ago and do not feel can be affecting us. Unfortunately, the fear we initially had of feeling these emotions—a fear as hidden from us as the emotion itself—prevents us from acknowledging this burden or even considering that it exists. Even when we are able to face these emotions, we don't know it.

Hypertension Beginning Decades Later

▸ Theresa, a slim and attractive fifty-four-year-old, was married to an executive at a large insurance firm. They had two children: a daughter, twenty-seven, and a son, twenty-nine. She was an interior design consultant.

Theresa's blood pressure had always been very normal, but her doctor found it to be elevated two years earlier during a checkup. She subsequently began taking medication.

At first, her blood pressure varied considerably. It could be 180/100, and an hour later, 110/75. Recently it had been more consistently elevated, averaging 170/100 when she checked it at home, despite the medication her doctor had prescribed. In my office, her blood pressure was 165–175/92.

Both her parents, who had died in their sixties, had had hypertension, as did her brother. However, her blood pressure had been perfectly normal for fifty-eight years, and then increased abruptly to a systolic blood pressure in the 170s. This pattern could not be explained by genetics alone, nor was there any recent stress to explain it. With this in mind I set out to find a possible explanation.

I inquired about Theresa's past and about how she got along with her parents. She answered that their relationship was so-so. Was she close to them? Not really. She told me she was always ambitious and energetic, never content to just "go along with the program." Because of this she was often in conflict with them. In a way she was the black sheep.

Did her father ever hit her? Yes, when he was angry at her, he punched her with his fist. Had he ever hurt her? Once he almost fractured the orbit of her eye. He apparently hit her whenever she did something that angered him, even if it was trivial. Her mother was intimidated and did not protect her. Her brother, who went along with the program, was not hit.

Theresa told me that she did not let this abuse affect her. She had her dreams. She had friends. She wanted to be an actress. She did well in school and took things in stride. Her spirit was not crushed or even dampened.

Along with the hypertension, Theresa told me she also suffered from migraine headaches, lifelong insomnia, and periods of recurring nightmares. The nightmares always had a similar theme. She was in a dark house and was scared. There was no one to protect her. She would wake up with her heart racing.

These problems, all unexplained, pointed me to a possible basis in hidden emotions. However, Theresa had recognized the injustice of her abuse and had distanced herself emotionally from her father, so I was not certain that this abuse was the cause of her hypertension.

I finally asked her if she had been sexually abused. She paused. Yes. She was forced to have sex with her father about twice a week from as early as she could remember, until she reached fifteen. She told me she had put this behind her as well. She never felt upset about it. No one knew of her past. She never told her husband, her friends, or anyone.

Once before, the issue of her sexual abuse had come up. She was depressed after her mother's death a few years earlier and saw a therapist, where the subject was raised. Therefore, she thought that she had dealt with it. She had not thought long about it, had shed no tears, and told no one else.

I suggested to Theresa that given her history and her migraine headaches, insomnia, and nightmares, I thought there was a strong possibility that hidden emotions from her past were relevant to her hypertension. I explained to her that I believed blocking out her emotions during her childhood had enabled her to get on with her life and avoid serious emotional consequences. However, the relevant emotions, even if forty years old, still lurked inside. With the strength and perspective of the adult, she could face the emotions that the child inside had avoided. Avoiding them was exacting a greater and greater price. Dealing with the past would mean feeling pain, but could be healing.

Looking at the entire picture, Theresa immediately grasped what I was suggesting. She was certain there was a link.

She returned a week later. Her blood pressure, checked at home, was normal, averaging about 120/75–80, still on medication. She felt better, less agitated. In my office her blood pressure was 145/90, improved, but still above normal. I discontinued her medication and her blood pressure remained in the 130s/75–85. The migraine headaches, nightmares, and insomnia that had plagued her for years ceased even before she began psychotherapy.

Theresa decided to see a psychotherapist experienced in treating victims of sexual abuse. Over several months, she would often return home from sessions in tears. She also came to realize how she had allowed herself to submit to the wishes of others her entire adult life, never seeing it as a problem or relating it to her past.

A year later, Theresa was still off all medication. Her blood pressure at home and in my office was normal.

Theresa's story did not end here. The emotional trauma had been extremely severe and prolonged, and at a young age. The real work of true emotional healing began a year after she first saw me, when some important, albeit not overwhelming, stresses triggered a bursting of emotions she could no longer hide. For weeks she cried, feeling the terror and horror she had been concealing. At fifty-nine, she was experiencing the emotions she fortunately had shut out as a child. She could now visualize her father, who had died several years earlier, and, in rage, scream at him: "How could you do this to a little girl?" She reminded me so much of Juan, except that the emotions were bursting through.

Although very independent her entire life, she needed a lot of support at this time, and got it. Theresa had never viewed her husband as capable of being emotionally supportive. She couldn't; she couldn't trust any man. She finally revealed her past history to him, and, to her surprise, he listened and was a bastion of support for her when she needed him. As it turned out, he had suspected the abuse for years, having seen her avoid any movie or television program that dealt with child abuse.

Theresa was also supported by her psychotherapist, with whom she had already established a relationship. The psychotherapist also prescribed paroxetene (Paxil), an antidepressant, to lower the intensity of the emotional storm. The emotional pain subsided, and she continued the very painful process of healing from the severe abuse of her past.

During the worst of her distress, Theresa's blood pressure temporarily rose to the 140s, a far milder elevation than that which she had had for two years when she was completely unaware of these emotions. It subsided without antihypertensive treatment. ◀

Theresa's story is not complete. Her healing process will require time and will not occur all at once. Nevertheless, she has already benefited greatly from the awareness she has gained.

Her migraine headaches, insomnia, nightmares, and hypertension have all improved. She feels much closer to, and trusting of, her husband. And, perhaps most important, she is able to view the emotional storm, which in light of her previous depression, was probably inevitable, as a healing process rather than as an unexplained depression—as emotional breakthrough rather than emotional breakdown.

ESSENTIAL HYPERTENSION should not begin abruptly. In the medical community, when it does, it generates an excited search for an unusual cause. Doctors may order a kidney scan, a Doppler sonogram of blood flow to the kidney, or an arteriogram to determine if the hypertension is caused by a narrowing of an artery supplying blood to either kidney. They may order blood and urine tests to detect a pheochromocytoma (a rare tumor that produces adrenaline and noradrenaline, as described in Chapter 7) or an inflammatory or other injurious process in the kidneys. Rarely, tests to look for a brain tumor may be needed.

However, the excitement quickly fades when the diagnostic tests come back negative, as they usually do. Treatment then consists of trying different medications to try to control the blood pressure. This is state-of-the-art treatment, altered somewhat as new medications are developed and marketed.

The question remains, however, Why does someone suddenly develop marked hypertension? When a person is clearly in the midst of extremely severe stress, the rise in blood pressure can be readily attributed to the stress. However, in most, stress or emotional distress does not provide the answer; without considering hidden emotions, an answer is rarely found.

An important and intriguing aspect of Theresa's hypertension was that it did not begin until decades after her abuse. The long interval obscured the relationship between the two. Uncovering the history of abuse, by itself, also did not prove its link to hypertension. It was the disappearance of her hypertension upon recognition of those emotions that confirmed the link.

The long interval without hypertension suggests that deeply buried emotions that are nowhere near conscious awareness might not affect blood pressure. The recent increase in Theresa's blood pressure suggests that these emotions were now closer to the surface of awareness. An analogy can readily be found in another late manifestation of trauma, post-traumatic stress disorder, which can first appear decades after an event.

Threatened by these emerging emotions, there were two paths Theresa could have taken. One was to continue to believe that there was no reason for her hypertension, migraine headaches, insomnia, or nightmares. This path would have required lifelong antihypertensive medication and possibly an endless battle against migraines and insomnia. The depression, which she had first experienced after her mother's death, was likely to have recurred. The cause of all these afflictions would have been viewed as unknown.

The other path, which she chose, was to consider the role of emotions she thought she had put behind her. This path was a painful one but provided the opportunity to heal, physically and emotionally. This is the path rarely taken because few realize that unexplained medical conditions can be linked to hidden emotions.

How Common Is Emotional Trauma?

At first I thought patients whose hypertension could be explained by old trauma were a rarity. However, I came to realize that emotional trauma, whose impact is often minimized, can be found in the past history of most people. It could be relevant in many people with unexplained hypertension.

How common is a history of trauma? In this assessment I believe it is important to start in childhood, where we are at our most helpless and delicate, and where, as a result, trauma can be the most overwhelming. People often overlook trauma that occurred during childhood because it happened so long ago. They might not even remember it as trauma and might not even remember that it occurred. They like to believe it faded away without affecting them, but the perceptions and emotions related to painful childhood events do not fade away.

The precise and persisting imprint of childhood experiences was illustrated to me as a medical student while I was observing the performance of a hypnotist. Part of his demonstration never faded from my memory. A twenty-five-year-old physical therapy student was easily hypnotized and was told that she was six years old. In response to questions, she answered that she was in second grade. She answered that Brooklyn, where she lived, was the capital of New York State (as an adult she knew that Albany, not Brooklyn, is the capital). "How much is two and two?" "Four." "How much is two times two?" "I don't know."

At six she knew how to add but not how to multiply. Her perceptions as a six-year-old lingered unchanged inside her. In the same way, emotions and perceptions related to painful events, even though seemingly forgotten, are retained, similarly unchanged by time.

In a study published in the *Archives of Family Medicine* in 1995, Peggy Wagner found a childhood history of some form of abuse in 66 percent of the adults she studied, including physical abuse in 39 percent, sexual abuse in 24 percent (among women), and emotional abuse in 55 percent. A history of abuse was associated with an increased likelihood in adulthood of psychological problems as well as physical problems such as chronic pain, stomach trouble, insomnia, sexual difficulties, fatigue, skin trouble, and poor health in general.

Charles Whitfield, in his book *Memory and Abuse*, reports that over half of the adult population has suffered physical, sexual, or emotional trauma during childhood. Harriet MacMillan reported in the *Journal of the American Medical Association* in 1997 that 13 percent of women reported a history of sexual abuse during childhood, including 11 percent reporting severe sexual abuse. Four percent of men reported a history of severe sexual abuse. Physical abuse and severe physical abuse were reported by 31 percent and 11 percent of men, respectively, and by 21 percent and 9 percent of women. These figures might underestimate the prevalence of abuse since they do not include those in whom memory of the abuse was also hidden.

MANY OF MY PATIENTS who have acknowledged a history of physical abuse view the beatings they received as stern discipline rather than abuse. Many consider the "discipline" they received as normal, because other children they knew were also beaten. Many mistake emotional abuse, which was even more common than physical or sexual abuse, for the fabric of normal day-to-day life. Yet even if, and perhaps especially if, unrecognized, it causes considerable damage.

People often overlook a history of childhood abuse because it does not trouble them as adults. Yet if the emotional trauma of a dysfunctional home, let alone overt abuse, can lead decades later to severe and persisting emotional manifestations, it is not hard to suspect that this often hidden burden can also lead to elevation of blood pressure and other physical manifestations.

In some instances of childhood abuse, the spectre is raised of false memory stimulated by the suggestion of a psychologist. Although this issue is important, I believe the relationship between childhood abuse and hypertension is real for a simple reason: The patients I have seen are not blaming anything on the abuse. On the contrary, they are saying the opposite, insisting that there was no lingering effect. They are not seeking revenge. Therefore, the abuse or trauma they recall is believable.

ABUSE BY FAMILY MEMBERS is not the only trauma to which children are subjected. Many are survivors of other trauma such as parental death or the increasingly common trauma of parental divorce. Traumatic events from outside the family, such as random violence, natural disasters, and war, are often particularly brutal in their suddenness and finality.

When you consider all these types of emotional trauma, it is apparent that many, if not most, adults have endured some traumatic experience in their childhood. The ability to block extremely painful emotions from awareness was a gift to children who would otherwise have been overwhelmed emotionally, particularly if facing these emotions by themselves. However, it still leaves the risk of long-term consequences.

PEOPLE ALSO SUFFER traumatic events in adulthood and block overwhelming emotions related to them. Fran Norris, in a study of a thousand people, reported in the *Journal of Consulting and Clinical Psychology* in 1992 that 69 percent of adults have experienced major trauma in their lifetime and 21 percent within the previous year alone. The most common events were the tragic death of a loved one, robbery, motor vehicle accidents, and physical assault.

Most researchers looking at the relationship between stress and hypertension focus more on current day-to-day stress than on more traumatic events that may have occurred years earlier. Yet I would suspect that the lingering effects of emotions related to the death of a child ten years ago, even if hidden, can affect blood pressure more than emotions related to current work stress. People tend to ignore old trauma, particularly when they don't feel distressed by it and have relegated it to the past. In this way, its relationship to hypertension is obscured.

Difficulties in Recognizing Trauma

I was first able to see the link between hidden emotions and hypertension when they were related to trauma that was overt and easily identifiable. However, as I continued on my path of discovery, I saw that overwhelming stress also comes in less dramatic guises, often not uncovered until I asked the extra questions.

I realized that the relationship between trauma and hypertension is not a straightforward one. I would like to be able to show that people who have hypertension experienced one or more of a short list of severely traumatic events. However, I cannot, because a much longer list of events that are potentially overwhelming occurs in the lives of almost everyone. Also, a given event will have a different impact on different people. One person might block emotions related to it whereas another might not. Some people, like Beverly, feel and discharge emotions related to losing a child, whereas others, like Leonard, do not. For some people, even events that would not seem severely traumatic can be overwhelming, depending on circumstances and personality.

The relationship between hidden trauma-related emotions and hypertension is also obscured by the effect of susceptibility to hypertension. Hidden emotions are much more likely to cause hypertension in someone who is genetically susceptible to it or who is obese than in someone who is not. In others, those emotions can lead to migraine headaches, asthma, colitis, or other conditions.

Another major barrier in recognizing the impact of old trauma is that it is often difficult to determine from what someone tells us that a given event was severely traumatic. The stories of two patients illustrate this dilemma.

> ▸ Peter, sixty-two, was on a high dose of four medications, yet his blood pressure was still very high, 170/110. He had retired after undergoing coronary bypass surgery eight years earlier. He had never married and was content living alone. He enjoyed the time he spent with his nieces and nephews. Money was tight, but he managed.
>
> I sought the reason for his stubborn, severe, and longstanding hypertension. He was not obese. He had no more stress than anyone else. Tests to look for medical causes of his hypertension, such as narrowing of the artery to his kidney, had been negative.
>
> Peter told me his mother died of pneumonia when he was one, and his father, unable to take care of five children, had placed all of them in an orphanage. He told me that life at the orphanage was okay and that his father had visited every week. He rejoined his father at home when he was fourteen.
>
> After struggling for a few months in an attempt to control Peter's blood pressure, I talked further with him about life at the orphanage. This time, with more questions, a different picture emerged.
>
> I asked him if he was ever hit.

Of course, but "that goes with the turf."

How was he hit and how often?

He said he was hit about once or twice a month. He could receive five or ten lashes with a belt. Or he could be ordered to stand still while punched by a counselor, priest, or nun. He said he was hit whenever his behavior was out of line, usually for trivial infractions.

Peter told me his sister was once pushed down the fire escape by a nun. Her back was broken and she had to be in a cast for three years.

Peter, not knowing any other childhood, did not feel his childhood was bad. He felt his job as an adult doing very mundane clerical work had been much more stressful.

Peter deplored how children today do not listen to their parents. He said he had not been like that. He had been raised "the right way."

Peter sees no connection between emotions and his hypertension. His current life is not particularly stressful and he sees no major problem in how he was raised. He sees no reason to think about those times, and feels no anger or sadness about the cruel and unfair beatings and terrorization that he accepts as having been good for him.

At this time there is no role for, and no possibility of, emotional intervention. Although I adjusted Peter's medication, his blood pressure varies from normal to very high. He remains on four medications. ◄

Peter insists he did not suffer an emotionally traumatic childhood. He does not believe his hypertension has anything to do with emotions.

► Tom, twenty-eight, five foot ten, slim and athletic, was in his last year of law school. He had been told of mild blood pressure elevation a few years earlier but had not paid attention to it. After suffering from headaches for several months, he saw his physician, who found his blood pressure to be extremely elevated at 190/130.

Tom was thin and was facing no major stress other than that felt by any law student. His mother had mild hypertension, but that could not explain why he had such severe hypertension at such a young age.

It is very unusual for a twenty-eight-year-old to have hypertension of this severity. In these cases doctors try hard to find a cause other than essential hypertension. We spend a fortune doing tests because we don't want to miss the cause.

Tom had the "million-dollar work-up." However, all tests were normal, leaving the unsatisfying diagnosis of essential hypertension. An ACE inhibitor (angiotensin-converting enzyme inhibitor, further described in Chapter 13) had no effect on his blood pressure. I treated him with a combination of a beta blocker (Tenormin) and an alpha blocker (Cardura), and his blood pressure improved.

Nevertheless, I felt uncomfortable. Why did he have such severe hypertension? Tom also wanted to understand why.

I looked for hidden emotions from the past. Tom's parents were living and he felt close to them. No abuse, no trauma. There was one possibly traumatic event: Tom's parents divorced when he was thirteen. Unfortunately, this could be considered "usual" stress, given current divorce rates. In addition, the divorce had been relatively amicable. Tom's parents remained friendly, shared joint custody, and were concerned with his reaction to the disruption of the family. As divorces go, it was not a particularly difficult one.

A year and a half after I first met Tom, his blood pressure was still a bit high despite the medication. I decided to inquire further about his past, looking for a clue of hidden, severely painful emotions.

As seems to happen again and again, a trivial question opened the door. I asked, "I assume your parents divorced because of the usual incompatibility and fighting."

"No. They always got along very well," he told me.

"You mean they were getting along perfectly well and then one day, out of the blue, they told you they were getting divorced?"

"Yes. I always thought we were the ideal family."

I asked Tom again about the aftermath of the divorce. He told me he had cried for a day or two and then "moved on." His mother asked him about his feelings. He never opened up to her. She sent him to a psychologist. He went for a few sessions and never opened up. Subsequently Tom was not upset or troubled, as he would be expected to have been. Not feeling the emotional pain, he did not have to resort to drugs or alcohol as an adolescent. He ended up on a solid career course. I discussed with Tom the likelihood that he had concealed very painful emotions in order to move on, and that the threat posed by those emotions and by his tendency to remain distant from his emotions could be playing a major role in his otherwise unexplained hypertension. Tom listened but was dubious. He was not interested in exploring this possible link to his hypertension.

Two years later he began to experience, for no apparent reason, insomnia and symptoms of anxiety and depression. He decided to begin psychotherapy. ◄

Although divorce hurts, the friction leading up to it usually provides some degree of forewarning. Sometimes divorce actually reduces tension. However, Tom was unaware of any problems leading up to the divorce. The facade of harmony had been maintained. Instead his "ideal" family was permanently torn apart overnight with no warning. In its suddenness, this divorce was likely to have been extremely difficult for him.

The impact of this seemingly well-handled divorce was also greatly magnified by Tom's tendency to hold in his emotions and to handle them alone. Emotional support was available and he needed it badly, but he was not the type to use it. He then had little choice but to conceal from himself emotions that were overwhelming him. The absence of the expected emotional distress was paradoxically a red flag, an indication that at the time he needed to block out the distress.

At the time Tom did better than most. Hiding away his emotions worked for him. He survived and thrived. However, I suspect his inattention to those and other emotions is at the root of the hypertension that developed years later.

In my first discussion with Tom, I did not uncover what made his parents' divorce unbearable: its suddenness. His every reply suggested that the divorce was not a severe trauma, yet a very different conclusion was available a year later. The difference hinged on my asking a single additional question.

Tom's story illustrates clearly why we cannot reduce the search for traumatic events to numbers and statistics. Parental divorce is very common. The stress is often severe, as manifested by the large number of children who end up with adjustment problems. In some cases, amicable, well-handled divorces make the distress less overwhelming. However, in Tom's case, I believe that the absence of any acknowledged effects belied the severity of the emotional impact. It is a mistake to believe that the emotional distress felt by a child, or reported later by an adult, is necessarily an accurate barometer of the true emotional impact of such events.

When I first saw Tom, and even a year later, he was not interested in exploring his past. Two years later he was. As I will discuss further in Chapters 11 and 12, the decision to explore the past is one that can only be made by the patient when he or she feels ready to do so. Psychotherapy begun prematurely is unlikely to cure hypertension.

In Tom's case, the ultimate proof is still missing: relief of his hypertension when he reconnects with his concealed emotions. However, he has begun the process of doing so.

MANY FACTORS CONTRIBUTE to how severely we are affected by emotional trauma: How old were we at the time of the event? Did we have a close-knit unit of family or friends? Were we able to confide our emotions in them? How much did the trauma alter our life? If a parent died, was the other parent lost to severe depression?

How expected or unexpected was the trauma? The sudden death of a parent is likely to be more devastating than the death of a parent after a long illness.

Did we learn from our parents how to obtain comfort from others, or did we learn to keep our emotions to ourselves, no matter how painful? What were our spiritual beliefs?

Finally, the severity of the event itself is, of course, a crucial factor. In some cases events are so devastating that hiding emotions might be the only means to survive and function. We blocked trauma-related emotions from awareness because we needed to *at the time*. We have every reason to be grateful for the capacity to have done so.

We would like to believe that, once hidden, these emotions will never affect us, but this is not true. They persist unchanged by time and do affect us. And, as stated by Bruno Bettelheim, "What cannot be talked about can also not be put to rest; and if it is not, the wounds continue to fester from generation to generation."

CHAPTER

When We Don't Know Our Own Emotions

I FIRST LEARNED TO RECOGNIZE the role of hidden emotions in hypertension in patients who reported a history of overt emotional trauma. Then I began to similarly recognize their role in patients without such a history. I gradually began to realize that, trauma or no trauma, it is isolation from our emotions and emotional isolation from others that has more to do with hypertension than does the day-to-day stress that we focus on.

When Calm Isn't Calm

▶ From the moment Donald entered my office, I felt very uncomfortable. It was a feeling not of dislike or impatience but of tension.

Donald was fifty, about five-ten, and perhaps slightly overweight, with thinning blond hair. His body language and pattern of speaking grabbed my attention. Every movement was a tense battle of muscles opposing muscles. His speech, similarly, was halting rather than flowing.

Although he was taking two medications, Donald's blood pressure had remained elevated. In my office, it was 145/95, mildly elevated, but apparently lower than his previous readings.

At the time I was not particularly focused on, or aware of, the role of emotional factors in hypertension. However, I found myself expressing to Donald my concern about the amount of tension that I sensed in him. I reassured him that we could probably control his blood pressure, but suggested he also address the tension. I urged him to consider consulting a psychotherapist. There was genuine urgency in my voice.

His reply astounded me: "I'm . . . not . . . tense. In . . . fact, . . . I feel . . . quite . . . relaxed."

I sensed that he was not kidding me or lying. He was telling me that he did not feel tense even though everything in his manner told me the exact opposite.

Donald worked in the garment industry and it was a busy and crucial time of year. I thought that could explain why he was so tense, but he said that business was no tougher than in other years and that he was not tense because of it. He told me he was happily married and was not under stress. He said, unconvincingly, that he would consider consulting a psychotherapist.

I saw Donald again a month later. He was feeling well and his blood pressure was 140/90, at the upper limit of normal. He still seemed very tense and still insisted that he wasn't. His wife, who had accompanied him at this second visit, supported my observations. She had been after him for thirty years to see a therapist. Donald agreed to do so, but said it would have to wait one more month until his busy season was over.

His wife called me two weeks later. Donald was dead. She had awakened that morning and found him lifeless. ◄

Donald most likely died a sudden cardiac death. However, he had not been a smoker. He had no family history of premature coronary death. He did not have diabetes or elevated cholesterol. Even though he had hypertension, he should not have had a heart attack at fifty. I had to suspect that his extreme tenseness had played a role in his death, even though he had insisted he did not feel tense.

SEEING PATIENTS LIKE DONALD indicates to me that people can be completely unaware of emotions written all over their face. I had always assumed that people who look very tense know that they are tense. I realized I was wrong. Although Donald's wife and I both saw him as extremely tense, he did not *feel* tense and could not understand why we thought he was tense. His death further suggested to me that the emotional distress that we don't feel might be very relevant to cardiovascular risk and to the discussion of mind–body medicine that surrounds us.

> ▸ Jimmy, sixty, a tall, white-haired, and very intense man, had been on medication for hypertension for twenty years. Recently, his blood pressure had been harder to control.
>
> Jimmy's mother had died when he was twelve. He does not remember how long he grieved, but he had managed to continue through the school year without any difficulty. His father became an alcoholic and was out of work for a while. It was Jimmy, not his father, who held the family together. Jimmy survived and succeeded.
>
> His wife described Jimmy as "a saint." Just like he did when he was younger, Jimmy took care of everybody. People came to him with their problems. He took care of his own problems by himself and never sought anyone's help.
>
> Whenever he came to see me, Jimmy looked worried. I asked him if he felt tense. He said no. He said there was no particular stress in his life.
>
> Jimmy remains on medication. ◂

Like Donald, Jimmy appeared tense while claiming he did not feel tense. His constant tension made sense only with the perspective of the childhood he described to me.

> ▸ Al, thirty-five, had severe hypertension. His blood pressure was usually above 170/120, no matter what medicine he took. He had been having headaches every day for six months.
>
> Al appeared easygoing; however, his life was not in great shape. Because of the headaches, he had to stop working. He was living off dwindling savings. His wife was threatening to leave him. (She eventually did.)
>
> I asked Al, given all this stress, how were his spirits? He responded genuinely that he was "as happy as a clam."
>
> Al remains on four medications. His blood pressure remains uncontrolled. ◂

Like Donald and Jimmy, Al insisted that he was not tense. Unlike them, he did not look tense. People will not see him as holding in his emotions but rather as being cool and calm.

A Different Look at Emotions

Studies of the mind–body link of hypertension have focused on the emotional distress we feel, which we sometimes "hold in." We might choose to hold in anger at our boss rather than express it. In such instances we know we are angry. Unable or unwilling to express anger against the person who provoked it, we might discharge it in other ways—some good, some not. We might lose our temper at our spouse. This might discharge the anger but will create a new stress. We might cope better by either playing basketball or commiserating with a friend. Or we might simply continue to feel angry until the anger eventually subsides. Although we might hold these emotions in and conceal them from others, they are not hidden from us. We feel them.

In talking about hidden emotions, I am talking about something very different. I am talking about emotions that we don't feel and don't even know we are hiding inside us. We don't *feel* angry at our boss even if friends think we should be infuriated. We might be very understanding, rationalizing that he is under extreme pressure, or that our performance merited his cruel rage. But we just don't feel angry. Similarly, in other situations, we might not know that we are tense or sad. We might insist we are relaxed, because we don't feel the tension inside us.

I see many patients who would respond on a psychological questionnaire that they are not tense or angry or depressed. If their life seems reasonably stable and they look calm and happy, their responses make sense. If their life is a disaster, or if they look very tense, the responses do not make sense. In other words, their responses have little meaning unless viewed in the context of their life circumstances.

Many people do not feel the emotion that is written all over their face. They would be shocked to hear that they are often perceived as angry or tense or sad, when they truly don't feel these emotions. In situations that can be expected to provoke emotional distress, they don't feel their distress and insist that they handle such stress very well. And they do handle problems without feeling upset.

Many other people, like Al, claim to be calm and also appear calm, no matter how much stress they are facing. Their appearance or facial expression tells nothing about what they harbor inside. It can be impossible to tell them apart from someone who is truly relaxed.

When someone always claims to be on top of the world, especially when events are not going his way, one has to wonder what emotions lie unfelt inside. As discussed by Jonathan Shedler in 1993 in *American Psychologist*, this is a major dilemma in mind–body research. Measuring what people feel does not take into account the strong emotions hidden inside. A person who harbors tremendous anger can honestly claim on a questionnaire that he does not feel angry, which I believe is why this research has not uncovered the link between emotions and hypertension.

How then can we tell if someone who looks calm is truly calm or harbors enormous anxiety or rage or sadness that he does not feel? It can help if we try to get a sense of the balance or imbalance between the stress someone is facing and the emotions he or she reports. When people are unaware of their distressful emotions, there is a mismatch between the amount of *stress* in their life and the amount of *distress* they report. I could not accept that Al was very happy, no matter how he looked, given the circumstances in his life.

Sometimes it is very hard to tell. Some people are aware of many of their emotions yet unaware in specific charged areas. Or they might feel one emotion but not another. Like Rhonda, whose story is told in Chapter 11, they might feel anxiety while hiding deep sadness or shame. Or they feel anger while hiding fear. Many hide major fears by focusing on aches or pains or fears concerning much more trivial problems.

We hide all kinds of emotions, such as anger, anxiety, fear, grief, sadness, helplessness, and shame. I don't know which is most closely tied to hypertension and suspect that any painful area of emotions can play a role, as long as we are engaged in a battle to not feel it.

Emotional Isolation: Living Alone with Our Emotions

I began to notice that people who tended to conceal emotions from themselves also tended to handle the emotions they did feel by themselves. Whether they lived alone or were surrounded by huge families, they never discussed difficult emotions with anyone. They were living in what can be called "emotional isolation," often without knowing it.

> ► Michael, thirty, was married with four children and worked long hours in an electronics store.
>
> He had already had a stomach ulcer. For the past two years, his blood pressure had been very labile, varying from normal to 180/110. On an ambulatory monitor, worn for twenty-four hours, it averaged 140/90, slightly elevated.
>
> He came to see me because he had had headaches for three days. His blood pressure, checked by a friend, had been 180/110. In my office, it was 144/86, mildly above normal, but not high enough to be the likely cause of his headaches.
>
> Michael wanted to know why he had the headaches and the hypertension. He looked very burdened but insisted that the stress he was facing was his usual stress—nothing more, nothing less. He worried about his wife, his children, and his parents, and he took care of a lot of people. Even so, he insisted he was used to it.
>
> I then asked what I have come to regard as a loaded question: Who takes care of you? Who do you go to when you are feeling a lot of tension?
>
> "I take care of myself."
>
> I suggested there might be a different way of handling the considerable stress in his life. He did not return to my office. ◄

Michael had learned the responsibility of taking care of others but had not learned to value taking care of, or even acknowledging, his own emotional needs. He was surrounded by people who loved him, yet he could not or would not confide his emotions in anyone. He could give care but couldn't receive it.

My words were foreign to him. Michael could not understand the dimension that was missing, or even realize it was missing. He is familiar only with handling his stress alone, and does not have the option of easing his distress by confiding it and receiving and accepting emotional support. Unable to do so and with no outlet for the tension trapped within, his only alternative is to struggle to hide it from himself. As the stress continues, his medical problems are likely to persist and to grow. Already he has headaches, hypertension, and ulcers.

Contrary to what Michael and many others might claim, I do not believe that day-to-day stress is the major cause of their hypertension. I believe it is the isolated way in which they are handling it, not even knowing there is another way. In their failing struggle to ignore what they are feeling, they end up with physical problems.

Michael's doctors will support his focus on his blood pressure and his physical symptoms, without ever recognizing or addressing the emotional isolation that underlies them. He will go from doctor to doctor, but it is unlikely that his medical problems or physical symptoms will end. His story is an all-too-common tragedy that need not occur.

Supermen and Superwomen: Superneglect of Our Own Needs

▶ Brad, thirty-four, is a wonderful man. He is a wonderful husband and a wonderful father to his four kids. He works long hours as an attorney, hoping to achieve partnership in his firm. He leaves home at seven in the morning and returns between ten and eleven at night. He works most weekends. He is also very active in community work.

Brad is a superman. He does for everyone. He is unselfish and unconcerned about his own needs—a perfect husband and father (when he is home), a perfect employee.

At thirty-four, Brad has severe hypertension and is on two medications for it. He does not see any problem that needs to be addressed. ◄

Brad is paying a price for being so wonderful. His blood pressure is telling us that even though he does not recognize it, the stress of his lifestyle is harmful and unacceptable.

I was not asking Brad to be selfish. I was asking him to restore a little balance in his life, to also pay attention to his own emotional needs rather than focusing only on the needs of others. I was asking him to listen to what his blood pressure was telling us, that something in his life was not right.

In the long run, Brad is likely to have more years to do more for others, if he takes care of himself. I hope he will someday realize that.

I SEE MANY SUPERMEN (and superwomen) in my office. They are bright and they are achievers. They are often workaholics. Although it is tempting, and an easy target, to blame their hypertension on long working hours, their hard work is not the problem. The need to prove their value and to please other people, without awareness of their own needs, is what is toxic. The overwork is only one symptom of that neglect. I tell them that I believe they deserve to treat themselves a little more kindly. They are likely to argue.

Patients will tell me that this is how they have always lived. Or that circumstances leave them no choice (sometimes there genuinely is no choice). Or that they're okay. They don't know how to stop, to pause and look within, or to seek some relief by confiding their concerns with others, as years follow into decades of self-neglect.

At some point the mind and body will protest. That is when physical symptoms and illness appear, such as hypertension, and it will generally be regarded as an entirely physical problem. Even when ill, they refuse to consider the mind or the self-neglect. Instead, with pills to keep patching their health together, the self-neglect is perpetuated. Their emotions are screaming at them, but they can't hear.

The Pros and Cons of Not Feeling
Our Unwanted Emotions

It is hard to assess what someone does not feel. If you feel relaxed, or up, most of the time, it does not mean that you are necessarily harboring a mountain of hidden distress. However, certain characteristics, some of which may dominate more than others, can suggest that you are concealing more than you suspect.

People who hide many of their unwanted emotions from themselves tend to be described as:

- ► Mr. Nice Guy
- ► Even-keeled
- ► Emotionally self-reliant
- ► Emotionally unavailable
- ► A model citizen
- ► An inflexible know-it-all
- ► A workaholic
- ► A superman or superwoman
- ► A person who insists he is not as tense or angry as he looks

Here is an exaggerated sketch to convey the flavor of the person who tends to unknowingly and routinely hide unwanted emotion. It describes a pattern that can be seen in men and women, and confers both advantages and disadvantages.

- ► He is often the solid citizen, an asset to his family and community. He might be the first to come to someone's aid.

He does things for everyone. He tries to please as many people as he can and does not complain about the heavy demands on his time and energy. He lets everything roll off his back. He ignores his own needs.

He tends to be even-keeled or might be jolly. He rarely feels down or moody. Even if he appears to others to be angry or tense or depressed, he insists he is not and cannot understand why people think he is. He insists things are okay, even when they are not.

He is very self-reliant. He does not need to lean on others for emotional support and doesn't even know how. In fact, others lean on him in times of crisis. He never shares his fears or sadness. He might share his concern about this ache or that pain, but not emotional pain. He learned in childhood to manage on his own.

He is a problem solver. He figures out what needs to be done and does it. His emotions don't get in the way. He is very pragmatic. He will talk about things and events more than about feelings. He might be very detail oriented.

He likes his routine and tries hard not to vary from it. He is most comfortable in familiar surroundings. In general, he does not like change. He will tell you he is who he is, period. He is not looking to change and believes people do not change.

He might be a workaholic. He will tell you he loves his work or that he cannot avoid the long work hours. He likes to keep very busy, even in his spare time. ◄

Many people who do not hide their unwanted emotions can also go through life without getting very angry or anxious about what many of us call the little things. They are blessed. Unlike people who are hiding these emotions from themselves, they feel their negative emotions but do not dwell on them. They get angry but don't stay angry. Sometimes things bother them. Sometimes they feel low. When they need emotional support during a crisis, they seek it and gain strength from it.

Men or women who habitually hide their emotions differ in that they might claim that almost nothing bothers them. They insist they can handle their problems by themselves and do not require a shoulder to lean on. They survive trauma and bereavement without feeling severe emotional pain, but forfeit the opportunity for emotional healing and the comfort provided by connectedness with an empathetic relative or friend. They do not know what such comfort feels like and don't seek it.

We admire people who appear unfazed by problems that would trouble most others. They seem to go through life unaffected by stress. If they are lucky and encounter relatively little stress, they might get away with it. Otherwise, the burden of blocking more and more emotions can eventually lead to problems.

People who avoid unwanted emotions in this way are fortunate in that they do not suffer from feeling tense or down, but they forfeit the guidance and healing that negative emotions provide. For example, it is tension that tells us to sit down with our spouse and deal with whatever conflict is causing it, before it escalates. If we feel that everything is okay, we are not motivated to deal with problems or make changes.

If we didn't learn that emotional distress is a useful signal, then we are unable to use it to reassess our values and priorities. Instead, we can only view it as something that we must avoid.

The overly even-keeled person can be very aware of reactions related to external, and minor, day-to-day problems, while hiding more difficult emotions. He may feel love and connectedness in as limited a way as he feels anger and anxiety. There is an inner emotional void that is filled with external details. Ironically, having never experienced more, he is unlikely to be troubled by, or aware of, those limitations.

Thus, there are advantages and disadvantages to being unaware of unwanted emotions. It spares us emotional discomfort, but stands in the way of change and accumulates a burden of hidden distress. Depending on the severity of the stress we encounter and our genetic makeup, this burden places us at risk of ultimately developing hypertension or other physical illnesses. Of course, when someone asks us what distressful emotions might underlie the illness, we will insist that we have no emotional distress and that emotional factors do not play a role.

Hiding Our Emotions: Its Roots in Childhood

We don't develop a pattern of hiding our emotions for no reason. This pattern is usually dictated by events and relationships in childhood. It evolved as the best way to survive in that early environment.

The manner in which we handle stress begins in childhood, in the family. Someone who hides his emotions is likely to have grown up in a family or situation where feelings were not discussed or confided. In other words, his childhood was marked by emotional isolation.

> ▶ Ralph developed severe hypertension when he was eighteen. At thirty-two, on a twenty-four-hour monitor, his blood pressure averaged 180/130. There was no major stress in his life.
>
> Ralph's father had an enormous temper. He was always shouting. His temper was terrifying to those around him. Ralph learned to not feel terrified. As he put it, he learned to let things roll off his back. Like so many others, he had no need to confide his emotions in anyone, because he never let anything get to him.
>
> Ralph insists that stress has nothing to do with his hypertension, because nothing bothers him. If he is holding anything in, he will tell you he is unaware of it. ◄

WE ACQUIRE OUR MANNER of handling emotions during childhood. We learn either to confide and share our feelings, or to bear them alone, and ultimately to hide them from ourselves.

Although genetic factors may also be involved, it is the environment created by our parents and others that largely shapes how we will handle our emotions. Rather than understand and empathize with our fears, perhaps our parents told us there was nothing to be afraid of, to stop being afraid, even though there was something very real to be afraid of. Did they allow our anger or give us the message that harmony is to be preserved at all times?

In an interesting article in 1992, Hans Steiner traced the origin of this style of hiding distress to families that rewarded conformity. In such families, there was little outward antagonism or conflict; conflict was not allowed.

In many families, the emotions of the parents receive attention, while the emotions and emotional needs of the children are ignored. A child in such a home learns to also ignore his own emotional needs. Was responsibility to others inculcated while the emotional needs of the child were ignored? Many people are imbued with a sense of responsibility that makes them the model citizens they are. But there is an imbalance; they are unconcerned about taking care of themselves.

There is a pervasive attitude that we must avoid painful feelings. As children we are taught not to cry. When facing genuine danger we are told there is nothing to worry about. This serves to leave us alone with our fear, leaving us with a choice of being overwhelmed or learning to block out fear, even before we have felt it.

A child can tolerate fear or sadness better if he can share them with, and be comforted by, a parent, grandparent, sibling, or anyone. Children are more resilient if they have an emotionally available caregiver. However, this contact is unavailable in many homes. Even without trauma, life is a series of minitraumas when a child faces all of his or her emotions alone.

I encounter many patients who describe a wonderful childhood home where food, shelter, and toys were provided, but where this essential contact was not. The child learns not to feel very painful emotions, without even realizing that he is not feeling them. He does not remember any other way of being.

The pattern of blocking out emotions might also stem from overwhelming trauma in childhood, such as abuse or losing a parent. People with stories like Peter's in Chapter 5 learned as children to block out unwanted emotions and relatedness. This pattern may then dominate further development.

The child who didn't learn to share his anxiety, anger, pain, or grief becomes an adult who does not share them. He learned to not feel his distress and, as an adult, similarly blocks out much of his emotional distress, not even realizing he is doing so.

Men or women who grew up learning to hide their emotions from themselves will not recognize that their hypertension or other unexplained physical illness could be linked to these emotions. They are likely to insist that their life is okay, regardless of the stress in their marriage and relationships. They are not lying. They have learned either to not see what is wrong or to not realize when or how much they are troubled by it.

The Growing Trail of Evidence

Even though hidden emotions cannot be seen or measured and their role in hypertension is not widely studied, a surprising amount of research provides support for their role in hypertension. This support only begins with the failure of studies to implicate the emotions we are aware of, which forces us to look beyond the limits of our conscious emotions.

I look with interest at studies that show the opposite of what researchers with no particular interest in hidden emotions had expected to find. Here are a few examples. In a study reported in 1988, Marilyn Winkleby sought to show that among 1,428 bus drivers in San Francisco, those who had hypertension would report feeling more emotionally distressed than those who did not. Instead, she found the opposite; they reported feeling less distressed. The Alameda County Blood Pressure Study (see N. O. Borhani, 1968) reported that people who rated a given stress as milder than objective measures of that stress had the highest blood pressure. Eugene Meyer reported in 1978 that people with hypertension reported lower levels of emotional distress than did people whose blood pressure was normal. Nancy Krieger reported in 1996 that African Americans who felt victimized by discrimination had lower blood pressure readings than those who did not.

These and many other studies have noted the same reciprocal relationship between feeling distress and blood pressure; the less the awareness of distress, the greater the blood pressure. Reviews fairly consistently indicate that hypertension is associated with the tendency to inhibit emotional awareness (see J. Sommers-Flanagan, 1989; and R. S. Jorgensen, 1996). They indicate that the distress, anger, or resentment that we feel is not what drives hypertension.

James Lynch's fascinating studies show that when people discuss a "hot topic," their blood pressure can soar even though they are completely unaware of any emotional discomfort. Lynch states in his book *Language of the Heart*:

> Several patterns began to emerge. One was the striking contrast between the external calm of many of the people we monitored and the magnitude of their cardiovascular reaction when they

spoke. Even while their blood pressure surged into hypertensive ranges, and their hearts began to pound rapidly, many of these individuals appeared absolutely calm, typically smiling as they spoke. . . . It appeared that the greater the cardiovascular change when one spoke, the less likely was one to report being aware of any internal changes whatsoever.

An interesting lesson can be learned from the severest form of essential hypertension, known as *malignant essential hypertension*. This condition, more common among African Americans, is as serious as the name connotes. Without treatment, it leads to kidney failure or death within months. The cause is still unknown.

If the anger and anxiety people consciously feel are strongly related to hypertension, I would expect it to be most evident in this form of hypertension. However, in my experience, people with malignant essential hypertension generally are not very angry or anxious or depressed. Those who grew up and continue to live amid the violence, neglect, and cruelty of the urban ghetto do not seem to feel, or complain about, the anger or despair. Instead, they have malignant hypertension. Blocking out such emotions was important to their emotional survival, but it might also be at the root of their hypertension.

Occasionally I do encounter very anxious people who have markedly elevated blood pressure readings. However, most turn out to have a milder degree of hypertension than seems apparent, with readings exaggerated by nervousness during blood pressure measurement. I am not saying that it is impossible to be a nervous wreck and have truly uncontrollable hypertension, but I am saying that it is the exception, not the rule.

MUCH OF PSYCHOSOMATIC RESEARCH in hypertension involves questionnaires that measure the emotional distress people feel. As I discussed in Chapter 3, people with hypertension do not differ from others in their responses.

Questionnaires cannot measure the emotions we do not feel, but a few do provide an indication of the tendency to habitually hide emotions. It is on these questionnaires that responses of people with and without hypertension consistently differ.

One such questionnaire is the Marlowe–Crowne Scale of Social Desirability (see D. P. Crowne, 1960). This questionnaire asks people whether they always adhere to desirable behaviors such as always telling the truth or never getting angry at anyone. People with high scores are claiming that they meet a nearly impossible standard. Daniel Weinberger reported in 1979 that people who tend to hide distressful emotions often have a high score on this scale in combination with a low score on anxiety questionnaires. Typically they will insist that they are not upset in situations that most people would find upsetting. A study by Jens Asendorpf in 1983 showed that such individuals, when confronted with laboratory stress, reported little anxiety, while their facial expression indicated the opposite. As Weinberger discussed in 1994, they are unable to acknowledge to themselves shortcomings that are universal.

Studies have found consistently that people with hypertension are more likely than others to have high scores on the Marlowe–Crowne Scale and similar scales (see M. A. Wennerholm, 1976; and W. Linden, 1983). In my own research, reported in the *American Journal of Hypertension* in 1996 and in the *Journal of Psychosomatic Research* in 1998, 51 percent of the seventy-four subjects who had hypertension, and an even higher percentage of those with severe hypertension, had high scores, compared to only 24 percent of the fifty subjects who did not have hypertension.

When such individuals are confronted with stress in the laboratory, they report less anxiety yet manifest a greater increase in blood pressure than do others (see A. King; D. A. Weinberger, 1979; S. Warrenberg, 1989; and J. B. Asendorpf, 1983). Studies using the Marlowe–Crowne Scale report similar findings in other physical conditions. Brenda Toner, in 1992, reported high scores in many people with irritable bowel syndrome. James Gross reported that high scores were common in cancer patients. Roger Dafter discusses how people with the tendency to hide emotions from themselves also have a reduced immune response. Perhaps because of this tendency, he found that women with breast cancer who feel the least anger and sadness do worse than those who feel the most. Such findings underline the need to look more closely at the role of hidden emotions in many disorders.

Who Develops Hypertension?

Although the tendency to hide emotions increases the likelihood of developing hypertension, clearly not everyone with this tendency ends up with the condition. My studies and experience with patients suggest that the likelihood of developing hypertension is affected considerably by four factors: obesity, family history of hypertension, the severity of stressful life events encountered, and whether we reach the point at which we can no longer hide from our emotions.

Obesity

There is wide agreement that obesity, defined as exceeding ideal body weight by at least 20 percent, is a risk factor for hypertension. In his review on the link between obesity and hypertension, Stephen McMahon suggests that obesity might be responsible for as much as 30 percent of hypertension. Rose Stamler reported in the *Journal of the American Medical Association* in 1978 that the risk of developing hypertension was doubled by obesity. Thus, someone who hides his emotions is more likely to develop hypertension if he is also obese.

Genetics

Ryk Ward, in a review published in 1995, concluded that about 20 to 40 percent of hypertension could be attributed to a genetic predisposition. It is suspected that there are many "hypertension genes," although none has yet been clearly linked to the development of hypertension. Meanwhile, until specific genes are linked to a predisposition to hypertension, the only way to tell whether or not you have a genetic predisposition is simply by your family history.

Someone who hides his emotions from himself is more likely to develop hypertension if he also has a genetic predisposition.

If instead he has a family history of asthma or other conditions, he might be prone to develop those conditions.

There is a tendency nowadays to blame many conditions entirely on genetics, and scientists have found a genetic link in alcoholism, depression, and other conditions that tend to run in families. However, this link is unlikely to be the entire cause of those conditions. We cannot ignore the mind–body relationship.

In some people with a genetic predisposition, hypertension might be entirely due to genetics. However, in many others, it is not. Even if you have a strong family history of hypertension, emotional factors can still be playing a large role in determining whether hypertension develops and how severe it will be.

In my experience, hypertension that is largely genetic is relatively easy to control with antihypertensive drugs, as I discuss in Chapters 10 and 13. When genetic and emotional factors are both involved, the resulting hypertension can sometimes be more severe and harder to control. When someone's blood pressure is very difficult to control, I usually find that hidden emotions are involved. So even if hypertension genes are identified, the role that emotional factors play in the severity and outcome of hypertension cannot be ignored.

The Severity of Stressful Life Events

▶ Clarence, seventy-two, could not tell me how long he had had hypertension. He never liked going to doctors and had rarely had his blood pressure checked. Finally, two years ago, he went to a doctor for a checkup and his blood pressure was elevated. Despite medication, his blood pressure remained very elevated, running about 160–180/90–100. In my office, and on an ambulatory monitor, it was 175/105. Blood tests indicated damage to his kidneys, suggesting also that he must have had the hypertension for a long time.

Clarence's hypertension did not make sense to him, because he was thin, neither of his parents had had hypertension, and his life was calmer than ever. He had retired after working on Wall Street for thirty years and did part-time consulting, which he enjoyed much more. He had never married and had no children. He had seen combat in World War II. I asked him about it.

Clarence told me that he had been in the infantry and had entered combat at a time when casualties were heavy. He guessed that at least 90 percent of the men he trained with were killed in battle.

At nineteen, his war experience had been terrifying to him. At one point, he was lost and afraid he would end up in German hands. He was so terrified, he even considered shooting himself. He ended up finding the American troops. Four days later he was wounded, in effect saving his life as he was removed from combat. Weeks later, recovered from the shrapnel wounds, he was back on the front, but in less dangerous conditions.

He returned home and went to college.

I asked Clarence if he had talked much about his war experience. Perhaps every decade or so it would come up in conversation. Had he ever talked with anyone about the terror he had experienced? No.

An only child in a middle-class home, Clarence was never hit or abused. His parents were not alcoholics. They were good parents. I asked him if he had ever discussed his war experience with them. No. They apparently had been very worried after receiving notification that he had been wounded. He told them about his wounds.

His physical wounds had been minor. The terror he had experienced was not. He never mentioned that aspect of his experience to them or to anyone. Instead his parents talked about how scared they had been.

I asked Clarence if as a child he had ever discussed his feelings with his parents. No.

Clarence was accustomed to being alone with his emotions and dealt with his war experience in the same way. At seventy-two, he is unlikely to alter the solitary way in which he handles his emotions, or to engage that which he hid long ago. His treatment will require lifelong antihypertensive drugs. ◄

Although Clarence says he feels relaxed and has no major stress in his current life, his history offers a mind–body explanation for his hypertension. Did he develop hypertension because of the blocked emotions related to wartime trauma? Or, as research psychologists might contend, did he develop hypertension because he tended from childhood to not feel or communicate unwanted emotions?

I believe either could be the explanation, or, more likely, a combination of both. Clarence's isolation from his emotions might not have led to hypertension had the burden of hidden emotions not included the wartime trauma. Similarly, the wartime trauma by itself might not have led to hypertension if it had been confided and comforted. Like Clarence, if someone tends to not feel his distressful emotions, he is more likely to develop hypertension if he has encountered severely stressful life events than if he has not.

I believe Clarence's story illustrates another dilemma in mind–body research. Does the emotional basis of hypertension lie in personality style or in the traumatic events we encounter? The answer is that neither can be considered in isolation from the other. This is why studies that focus only on personality or only on traumatic life events, but not both, cannot unravel the mystery of hypertension. Neither obtains a full picture of the individual.

When We Can No Longer Hide from Our Emotions

I encounter many patients who reach a point where it has become harder and harder to keep their unwanted emotions out of awareness. The burden of hidden emotions might be too great, or the defenses keeping them from awareness might have weakened. In some, recent events might have aroused long-dormant emotions. Whatever the reason, the battle to keep those emotions hidden, itself waged without any awareness, becomes a greater and greater internal crisis.

The crisis might be physical, with bouts of unexplained severe hypertension or headaches, chest pain, fatigue, insomnia, or any other disruptive physical symptom. The syndrome of unexplained episodic hypertension, described in the next chapter, is one such crisis. The crisis could alternatively be an emotional one, with unexplained anxiety or depression. In some people, both emotional and physical elements are present.

When such medical crises appear, a search for a physical cause is needed and is conducted. However, when none is found, it is increasingly likely that hidden emotions are involved.

Such crises can be difficult to manage but can turn out to be an opportunity for awareness and healing. They have become a turning point in the lives of some of my patients, as I'll discuss in Chapters 11 and 12.

When bouts of unexplained hypertension or other unexplained conditions are viewed and treated as a purely medical problem, this opportunity is lost. Patients are left with a condition that will rear its head again and again, whose cause will not be understood, and which might require medication for a lifetime.

In my experience, these physical crises are telling us that the old order is falling apart, that hiding from ourselves is not working. Like Rhonda, whose story is discussed in Chapter 11, we can fight to retain the old order, but it is usually a losing battle.

THE INTERPLAY of the stressful life events we have encountered, of how we have handled them, our genetic predisposition to develop hypertension, and our body weight all contribute to whether hypertension develops and how severe it is. Neither obesity nor genetics nor emotional factors alone can explain the entirety of hypertension. All must be taken into consideration.

In a study I reported in the *Journal of Psychosomatic Research* in 1998, the tendency to not feel unwanted emotions was a greater risk factor for hypertension than was obesity or family history. I also suspect that in people with severe hypertension, a condition that neither obesity nor genetics comes close to explaining, hidden emotions are the most important contributing factor.

The Enigma of Episodic Hypertension

7

ONE OF THE MOST DRAMATIC and disabling forms of hypertension that I see is the syndrome of episodic hypertension. People with this form of hypertension suffer sudden and unexplained episodes of severe blood pressure elevation, usually accompanied by severe physical symptoms such as headache, chest pain, or shortness of breath. Strikingly, between episodes the blood pressure is normal or near normal in most people.

I have seen dozens of patients with this condition, most of whom have seen numerous physicians without finding an explanation or effective treatment. However, looking at hidden emotions has opened the door to an explanation in almost every single case and has led to the only explanation that thus far makes sense of this disorder. More importantly, this understanding has led to successful treatment in many patients, and, in some cases, to a cure. My findings concerning this syndrome were published in the journal *Psychosomatics* in 1996 and in the *Archives of Internal Medicine* (in press).

A Medical Mystery

► For seven long years, Vera, fifty-one, had suffered episodes of severe hypertension. She had received no explanation for them and no effective treatment.

Her attacks always seemed to occur out of the blue and would then follow a predictable pattern. She would awaken from sleep with sweating, dizziness, tingling, weakness, and a severe throbbing headache in the back of her head. If she checked her blood pressure, it would be about 200/120. During the attacks she felt extremely sick and weak, and was in too much pain to function.

The attacks occurred every few weeks and lasted anywhere from a half hour to twelve hours. Her blood pressure would then fall to normal, leaving her exhausted. Her blood pressure between attacks was 145/90 or lower.

Because of the severity, frequency, and unpredictability of the attacks, Vera's life had effectively drawn to a halt. She had to quit her job, could not plan any trips, and was always living in fear of the next attack.

She had not been passive in seeking treatment. By her count she had seen thirty-nine physicians, including specialists at numerous major medical centers. She had had every relevant diagnostic test and had tried various antihypertensive medications to no avail. ◄

Vera's history fit the classic textbook description of a *pheochromocytoma* (which we'll call a "pheo," for short). A pheo is a tumor of the adrenal gland, usually nonmalignant, that secretes adrenaline and noradrenaline into the bloodstream, causing episodes of severely elevated blood pressure. The blood pressure can be sky-high during attacks yet entirely normal at other times.

A history such as Vera's always provokes testing for this rare and dangerous but usually curable tumor. Blood and/or urine tests can diagnose it by documenting high levels of adrenaline or noradrenaline or their metabolic products. An MRI (magnetic resonance imaging) and sometimes other scans are then performed to locate the tumor itself.

Physicians immediately suspect a pheo in patients with episodic hypertension. However, few patients actually have this tumor. Once a pheo is excluded, a cause for the symptoms is rarely found.

Medical researchers love to study pheos, investigating the hormones they secrete, and the blood tests and scans that can diagnose and locate them. In the past fifty years, there have been hundreds of scientific articles about this rare tumor. Ironically, there are only a dozen or so articles about the much greater number of people who are suffering from episodic hypertension but do not have a pheo. It is as if no one is interested in this fascinating mystery. The few articles that have been written have not come up with a cause or treatment.

▸ My first task in seeing patients like Vera is to seek a medical cause, particularly a pheo. In Vera's case, my task had been simplified. She had already had every test imaginable and none had suggested a pheo or any other cause. It made little sense to repeat the tests again.

I prescribed a combination of antihypertensive medications to somewhat reduce the peak blood pressure during attacks. I also suggested to Vera that after seven years of visits to thirty-nine physicians it was increasingly unlikely that we were going to uncover a medical cause. I suggested that she consider the possibility of an emotional basis.

Vera felt her life was rather free of stress, except for her medical condition. We both agreed that minor emotional distress could not be blamed for such severe attacks. Therefore, in seeking an emotional cause, a search for hidden emotions was the only path left.

She described her childhood as "ordinary." There was no physical or sexual abuse, no parental alcoholism or drug abuse. She had been an only child, not particularly close to her parents. Her father had had a stroke when she was sixteen and was depressed until he died when she was twenty.

His illness and death had provoked little reaction because she never felt particularly close to him. In talking with Vera, I sensed a childhood of little emotional involvement. No stress, no distress. Everything was okay.

Vera seemed to keep many of her feelings to herself, or perhaps from herself. Since no medical explanation could be found, I felt there was nothing to lose by exploring this emotional angle: the possibility that unfelt distress within her was at the heart of the disorder.

I suggested this to Vera. Even if she disagreed with me, she had nowhere else to turn. The next physician was unlikely to find something thirty-nine others had not found.

Vera's reaction typifies the dilemma when physical illness has its origin in hidden emotions. Vera was not interested in pursuing an emotional cause because her symptoms were physical, not emotional. However, out of desperation she reluctantly followed my advice. She made an appointment with a psychologist, still proclaiming that there was nothing wrong in her life other than her medical illness.

With the psychologist's help, Vera was quickly able to see how she usually dealt with conflict by hiding her emotions from herself and not being upset. She came to see why she always felt there was no stress in her life. She had had little conflict with her husband because she had always been willing to ignore her own feelings.

This pattern of ignoring her feelings could be traced back to her childhood, when her feelings were ignored by her parents. She had learned to deal with distress that was never comforted or respected by a parent by not feeling it. As she described it to me later, she had been an "orphan with two parents."

Within three months, the attacks ceased. She had one attack eighteen months later, and then none in the five years after that. After seven years of medical tests, treatments, and unrelenting attacks, the syndrome had responded quickly to a talking therapy. She is better able to recognize her feelings. She asserts herself with her husband and feels like a different person from the woman she had been. And she is free of the fear of when the next attack will come. ◄

Many people experience a sudden and often considerable rise in blood pressure during moments of emotional distress. However, the syndrome I am describing here is very different. People with this syndrome insist that episodes are not related to stress or to feeling nervous. They typically describe the episodes as occurring out of the blue, often when they feel very relaxed.

During episodes, they feel very sick. The episodes can last for hours, leaving them drained of energy afterward for as long as a day or two. The syndrome is genuinely disabling.

It resembles panic disorder in that it occurs unpredictably, cannot be explained by current stress, and is associated with a variety of physical symptoms. It differs in the absence of panic and in the severe elevation of blood pressure.

The first few times I saw patients with this syndrome, I had no inkling of what caused it. The absence of emotional distress at the time of attacks had initially discouraged me from considering an emotional basis. However, I started to notice a pattern that offered a clue. One patient had been physically and sexually abused as a child. He insisted that the abuse had no lingering impact. Another was a Holocaust survivor. She also insisted it had no lingering emotional impact.

▸ Joe, thirty-five, was disabled for five years by attacks during which his blood pressure could rise to 250/140. He had been hospitalized in intensive care units several times, but extensive testing had not uncovered a cause. Combinations of many antihypertensive medications had failed to prevent the attacks or to control his blood pressure during them.

He reported no major stress other than his illness. He acknowledged having been beaten regularly as a child by his father, even when he behaved. None of his brothers were hit. The beatings had stopped when he turned sixteen.

I asked Joe how he felt now toward his father. He said he loved him very much. Any anger? Absolutely none. The past is past.

Joe was like a teddy bear. He felt no anger, anxiety, or panic. Nevertheless, treatment with the antidepressant amitriptylline (Elavil) and the antianxiety drug alprazolam (Xanax), a combination used for panic disorder, quickly eliminated his hypertensive attacks. ◂

I began to look more carefully at the past history of other patients who insisted that their illness had nothing to do with emotions or with their past history. In most I found a history of severely stressful events—events that they insisted had no lingering impact.

Not feeling emotional distress, many refused to believe that there could be an emotional basis. However, the response to emotion-based intervention, after years of failed medical treatment, offered the most compelling evidence.

► One patient of mine, Maria, an attorney, had grown up in a loving middle-class home in South America and insisted there had been no abuse. However, at forty, she had been suffering for three years from both muscle weakness and hypertension. For six months she had been suffering from unexplained bouts of severely elevated blood pressure. She had already seen physicians at several prominent medical centers. One had diagnosed chronic fatigue syndrome and had prescribed salt tablets, which only made her feel worse.

She did not describe any history of trauma, but because she had this syndrome I asked further questions. She mentioned that she had spent a month in jail as a political activist during her college days in her native country. I asked for more details. She then described how she had been blindfolded the entire month, beaten and tortured, told repeatedly she would be executed (and many of her friends were executed), and forced to sign confessions while blindfolded. She had put this experience behind her, never feeling any emotions related to it.

Because of the severity of Maria's trauma and the duration and severity of her physical symptoms, I felt that this was not the time for emotional probing. Instead, I recommended treatment with drugs, as described later in this chapter, using an alpha blocker and beta blocker for her hypertension, and an antidepressant and anti-anxiety drug to eliminate her attacks. Her physical condition improved rapidly. When she and her psychiatrist feel she is ready, she will begin the process of healing from her deep emotional wounds. ◄

Some might call Maria's syndrome a panic disorder, albeit without panic, or a post-traumatic stress disorder rather than episodic hypertension. I believe all these disorders are various manifestations of the same problem: survivors of emotional trauma struggling internally to keep hidden emotions out of awareness. Maria had been futilely seeking care for her physical disorder for three years. It remained a mystery until the mind–body connection of hidden emotions was considered.

HAVING FOUND AN EXPLANATION in hidden trauma-related emotions in many patients with this disorder, I began to also find an explanation in hidden emotions in a smaller number of people with the syndrome who, like Vera, had no history of conspicuous trauma. In them I found a lifelong pattern of hiding emotions, as I've described in Chapter 6. They insisted that they were fine, no matter what problems existed. In many of them as well, treating the disorder based on this understanding produced results.

What causes the sudden blood pressure surges that occur in this disorder? There is only one possible source—the sympathetic nervous system and the brain, whose role I will discuss in more detail in Chapter 13. As I reported in *Psychosomatics*, blood samples drawn during attacks revealed a dramatic increase in the level of noradrenaline, indicative of a massive sympathetic nervous system discharge. I believe this discharge is part of the internal and unfelt struggle to keep these unwanted emotions out of awareness.

What is most interesting is that the syndrome can develop decades after traumatic events, or after decades of habitually hiding emotions. The delayed appearance of this disorder resembles the delayed onset of Theresa's hypertension, which, as described in Chapter 5, developed decades after her abuse and resolved with recognition of that hidden burden. The long interval before these manifestations appear also is an important reason for the difficulty in realizing the mind–body link at the core of this disorder.

Finally, why does the battle against feeling hidden emotions manifest as sustained hypertension in some people and as episodic hypertension in others? I don't know the answer.

Drug Treatment

My experience tells me that most people with this syndrome can be successfully treated and can return to a normal life. Some, like Vera, can gain awareness of the emotions underlying the disorder, and the attacks will cease promptly when they do so. In others, with many layers of deeply painful emotions, this might take longer.

Some people with this disorder will consider psychotherapy. Others will not, either because they don't have emotional symptoms, or because they are not able or willing to face the deeply painful emotions they are hiding. Even in them, the right combination of medications can reduce or eliminate the attacks, as illustrated in the following two case histories.

> ► Frank, sixty-eight, ran a large textile factory until daily hypertensive episodes, which left him exhausted and unable to concentrate, brought his life to a halt. A combination of three antihypertensive drugs could not control his blood pressure.
>
> Frank had always been a tough guy; nothing fazed him. Seven years earlier his only son had been critically injured in a car accident. He survived but remained permanently paralyzed. Frank acknowledged that he loved his son very much. I said to Frank: "Yet you never shed a tear after the accident." "That's right," he responded.
>
> At sixty-eight, Frank was not interested in psychotherapy or "changing who I am." However, because I strongly suspected that hidden emotions were at the root of his illness, I prescribed a combination of an alpha blocker and a beta blocker (see Chapter 13 and the Appendix), to block the effects of the sympathetic nervous system on his blood pressure, and a combination of desipramine (Norpramin), an antidepressant, and lorazepam (Ativan), an antianxiety drug, to eliminate the attacks. His attacks ceased, his blood pressure returned to normal, and he went back to running his business. ◄

I do not believe that antihypertensive medications by themselves would have ever brought a halt to Frank's recurring hypertensive attacks. However, he was restored to a normal life once the hidden emotions causing them were addressed with medication.

> ▶ Phyllis, seventy, was a once divorced, happily remarried homemaker in an affluent suburb. Tests had not revealed any cause for the almost daily hypertensive episodes that had left her exhausted and homebound for the previous year. Antihypertensive medications had been unhelpful.
>
> She did not fit the popular stereotype of the battered wife, yet for years she had been victimized while married to her first husband. Although she said they loved each other very much, he hit her on many occasions, often with no warning. They had had no communication for years after their divorce, but he had begun to contact her shortly before the episodes began.
>
> Phyllis did not believe that her history was relevant to the disorder and did not wish to pursue it. Nevertheless, treatment with alpha and beta blockers, desipramine (Norpramin), an antidepressant, and clonazepam (Klonipin), an antianxiety drug, gradually brought a halt to her disabling hypertensive attacks and enabled her to resume all of her activities. ◄

I believe that acknowledging the hidden emotions at the root of this disorder, feeling them and dealing with the impact they have had, can lead to both physical and emotional healing. However, many people, like Frank, are unable to delve into their feelings. Others are very reluctant to delve into the past or into what they are not feeling. They usually are not aware of their fear of these emotions and instead tell me that they feel the past has nothing to do with their illness. Some simply don't return to my office, even though no other approach has helped them.

Some who are elderly or who have survived severe trauma often cannot be expected to address the hidden emotions. Fortunately, even without doing so, many can be restored to a normal life with medication, as long as it addresses the roots of the disorder.

To reduce the severity of the blood pressure swings, I prescribe a beta blocker, such as atenolol (Tenormin), combined with an alpha blocker, such as doxazosin (Cardura) or terazosin (Hytrin). In combination, they block the effects on blood pressure of sympathoadrenal discharge (see Chapter 13). Because the blood pressure is normal between attacks, I often prescribe modest doses, with extra doses taken at the time of an attack.

These drugs can reduce the severity of the attacks but often do not prevent them. If necessary, I also prescribe an antidepressant drug, such as desipramine (Norpramin) or paroxetene (Paxil), possibly in combination with an antianxiety drug, to abolish or greatly reduce the frequency of attacks. These drugs can largely eliminate attacks in most people with this disorder.

The Search for Clues

Having seen many patients with this syndrome, I believe a basis in hidden emotions can almost always be found. Therefore, if you have this syndrome, even if you cannot readily see a basis in hidden emotions, I believe it would be extremely worthwhile to consider the treatment options I have discussed.

As I write this chapter, there is still no other accepted explanation for episodic hypertension. If you have this condition and no cause has been found, even if you are certain that emotions are not involved, I urge you to consider the role of emotions that are not apparent to you and the treatment options available to you. Your life does not have to be put on hold any longer.

The Fate of Hidden Emotions

8

IF HIDING UNWANTED or overwhelming emotions erased them completely from our brain, as many would like to believe, it would be a wonderful way of dealing with them. Unfortunately, hiding them does not erase them. They persist within us, even if we don't feel them.

Even without erasing them, if hiding such emotions kept us free of their physical and emotional consequences for the rest of our lives, it would still be a wonderful solution. However, even though hidden from us, these emotions affect us, either subtly or overtly, whether right away or only decades later.

Are there people who can encounter traumatic events, feel the emotional distress, and recover without emotional or physical consequences? Yes. Suzanne Kobasa, in 1983, described the qualities of such hardy people. They tend to believe that they can at least partially control events. They regard change as a challenge rather than as a threat. They evaluate events in the context of an overall life plan. Their sense of purpose and involvement in life mitigate the disruption. They see in painful events the opportunity for personal development.

However, in coping with severely traumatic life events, particularly during childhood, most people do hide considerable emotion. Hiding such emotions protects us at the time, and we would be in great trouble if we were unable to do so, as discussed by Robert Lazerus in *The Costs and Benefits of Denial*. However, hiding them also leaves the risk of consequences later on.

Closing the Door on the Past

▶ Since she was twenty, Greta, now fifty-five, had severe and uncontrollable hypertension. Her blood pressure was often as high as 240/130. She had suffered side effects from many drugs, further hampering her treatment.

Greta is a vivacious, bubbly woman. She is married, has two children, and runs a small jewelry business. She claimed she had no major stress. She acknowledged that she occasionally boiled over, a hardly uncommon trait.

There was no obvious medical or emotional explanation for her hypertension. She had severe essential hypertension.

However, her past offered an answer. Her childhood in Poland had been interrupted by World War II. She and her family were displaced after her father was conscripted for military service. When she was fourteen, her mother, severely depressed, committed suicide.

Greta ended up in America and put the past behind her. Coincidence or otherwise, she has had severe, unexplained, and lifelong hypertension. She is not interested in dealing with the past. Her hypertension remains difficult to control.

Unlike Greta, her sister was depressed her entire adult life and ultimately also committed suicide. She never had a blood pressure problem, despite her life of unending and overwhelming distress. ◀

Looking at these two sisters, severe hypertension was clearly the more benign outcome. If it could be controlled with drugs, it would seem best to leave sleeping dogs lie, particularly in view of the severe nature of the trauma. Even if it cannot be controlled, a person unprepared or unwilling to deal with the past should not be coerced to do so.

▶ At forty-two, George's blood pressure was high, about 170/100. There was no current stress to explain it. He enjoyed his work as a biochemist. He said he had remained single because he was afraid of being abandoned by a woman.

His past revealed a very different life. At seven, in his native Vietnam, he was hospitalized because of starvation. At ten, he and a brother were sent to live in New York with an uncle because his parents could not afford to feed them. He was not to see his parents again for twenty years. After a year, his uncle vanished, leaving George and his brother on their own. George survived and ended up with a college degree, a career, and hypertension. His brother, who suffered a severe nervous breakdown, does not have hypertension.

When I asked George if he thought his past history might be affecting his blood pressure, he said no. He replied that his history was "no different than anyone else's." His certainty that the past was irrelevant, that it had no lingering impact whatsoever, was a telltale clue to me of considerable hidden emotion related to it.

George did not come to me seeking psychological help. Although healing from the past might help him reduce his blood pressure and perhaps help him enter into a committed relationship, he was not interested in facing those emotions. Perhaps someday he will. Or perhaps he knows best, and, no matter what the cost, should not attempt to explore those emotions. ◄

George is living a life well beyond his most optimistic childhood dreams. He does not wish to look at the past, even with the perspective and strength of adulthood. Perhaps he is unknowingly protecting himself from emotions that he truly cannot tolerate, concerning the starvation, the sudden separation from both parents, and the tender years on his own in a foreign country with a brother who fell apart. Having witnessed his brother's breakdown likely magnifies his fear of the emotions lying within.

CURRENT STRESS COULD NOT EXPLAIN Greta's or George's marked hypertension, but trauma from decades ago could. Blocking emotions at the time had helped both survive. The sister or brother who could not block them paid an enormous emotional price. Notably it was the sibling who managed to block off the emotions who ended up with the hypertension.

In my experience, people with hypertension, particularly severe hypertension, tend more often to be the survivors of their family rather than the emotional victims. They survived because they blocked off their emotions when they needed to, either during trauma or during a childhood marked by emotional isolation. This is why people whose hypertension is linked to emotions are less likely than others to occupy the couches of psychoanalysts, or to be on medication to help them control their emotions, because they have defended themselves from the emotions that would have troubled them.

However, although hiding these emotions served them at the time, it left a debt that can eventually affect them, physically or emotionally, at any time later in their life. In many, this hidden burden can be confronted and healed when life is more settled, even if it is decades later.

Physical Versus Emotional Consequences

Once we have hidden emotions, our defenses battle to keep them out of our awareness the rest of our lives. As Freud wrote: "The process of repression [hiding emotions] is not to be regarded as an event which takes place once, the results of which are permanent. . . . The repressed [hidden] exercises a continuous pressure in the direction of the conscious so that this pressure must be balanced by an unceasing counterpressure." Being unaware of emotions is not just a passive condition. It is maintained by continuing to actively, albeit unknowingly, block awareness.

The ultimate fate of these hidden emotions can vary. In some people, they remain locked away, deeply buried, for a lifetime seemingly without overt emotional or physical consequences. Even here, consequences such as dysfunctional relationships or insomnia may be viewed either as part of normal day-to-day life or simply accepted as unexplained.

Unfortunately, over time, the intrapsychic battle to keep these emotions out of awareness can take a larger and larger toll. Eventually it can affect us either physically or emotionally, or both, without our even knowing that we are engaged in this battle. The disorders that result cannot be explained by current stress and will persist unless their source in hidden emotions is recognized.

If our defenses allow the emotional distress to leak through into awareness, we will be subject to emotional distress whose source is unknown to us, with disorders such as anxiety, panic, or depression. Even if the disorder was triggered by an obvious recent event, focusing on that event does not lead to understanding or cure. Because of the emotional distress, people with these manifestations are likely to seek help from psychotherapists.

On the other hand, people whose defenses continue to keep out emotional distress end up with physical manifestations, such as hypertension or other unexplained medical disorders. Since they do not feel the distressful emotions, they might never suspect an emotional origin, and they seek help from physicians rather than psychotherapists.

The success of drugs in treating both physical and emotional disorders has reduced the interest in searching for their emotional basis. However, drugs do not cure, they often do not fully control the condition, and they often cause unwanted side effects. That is why understanding the basis in hidden emotions is not merely of theoretical interest. However, this path of understanding is rarely pursued, as patients and physicians alike continue to regard the origin of such disorders as unknown.

WHEN A PERSON'S SYMPTOMS or illness is physical rather than emotional, when she insists that emotionally she feels fine, it is difficult to consider the role of emotions that she is not feeling. This is precisely why the importance of hidden emotions in physical illness has eluded and continues to elude attention.

The most difficult step for people who are unaware of these emotions is merely considering that emotions they are *not* feeling are affecting their physical or emotional health. It is much easier to blame hypertension on lesser and temporary problems that *are* bothering us, such as work stress or a fight with a brother-in-law. However, distress from such problems rarely causes hypertension, and addressing this distress rarely cures it.

My experience suggests that when a person is able to recognize that he or she is affected by emotions hidden inside, physical and emotional healing are possible. This recognition, by itself, can have a dramatic impact on hypertension and physical symptoms, although true emotional healing does not occur that quickly.

Why the Link to Hypertension Is Difficult to See

Another reason we fail to consider the relationship between hidden emotions and hypertension is that in many ways the relationship is not a simple or straightforward one. As I've discussed, decades may pass before physical manifestations appear. Also, hypertension might not develop if someone is thin and has no genetic predisposition; other conditions might develop instead.

To some extent, we all hide emotions and resist feeling them, yet we do not all develop hypertension. The severity of the painful emotions we have hidden, the extent to which we habitually hide our emotions from ourselves, and the strength and inflexibility of the defenses we use all play a role in whether we are affected physically or not.

Another reason we fail to understand the impact of hidden emotions is that if we remember the facts of prior abuse or trauma, we mistakenly believe we are in touch with the painful emotions related to them. Often we do not realize that we can remember events in great detail while hiding the emotions related to them. We can remember events as if remembering the tragic tale of a boy whose story we read in a book rather than the story of our own life.

The relationship of hidden emotions to the physical manifestations they cause is a complex one. However, given the toll of so many conditions, whose cause and cure remain a mystery to us, we can no longer afford to ignore their role.

Why Now?

I am often asked why the burden of long-hidden emotions raises its ugly head when it does. The answer is not always clear, but several factors do make some sense of it.

In some people the hypertensive process does begin right after painful trauma. However, it might not be noticed because the blood pressure rise is gradual and does not eclipse the arbitrary figure of 140/90 until many years later, seemingly unrelated to the events that initiated it long ago. A person's blood pressure can be 130/85, rather than 110/70, and can be considered normal, even though it is 20 millimeters higher than it otherwise would have been.

In many others, as I've already discussed, blood pressure may remain truly normal for decades and then rise. This too makes sense. With time or age or accumulated stress, as cracks develop in our defenses, physical or emotional consequences ensue, regardless of current life circumstances. This is why hypertension and other disorders can appear in our thirties and forties, or later, even if our life circumstances are better than ever.

In many people, over time, the threat of those emotions can be more easily triggered. Often it is a trivial event that causes them to stir. For example, in Martha's story in Chapter 5, the trigger to her recall of being raped was the resemblance she noted between her cousin and the uncle who had raped her. A triggering event can often be so trivial it can be easily forgotten, contributing to the mystery of what is seen as new illness.

Another important trigger is unoccupied time. Many people avoid hidden emotions for decades by always being busy. How often do we hear of the empty nest syndrome after grown children leave home, or of depression following retirement or a period of restricted activity?

Ironically, hypertension or other unexplained physical conditions often appear when things seem to be at their best. The cracks in our defenses might simply be a result of age and time. Even so, when our lives are stable, we have a greater capacity to face, and heal from, emotions we previously needed to block out. We have the opportunity to shed defenses that we once needed, but now no longer need. However, just as ironically, we are usually our least introspective at times when our lives are going well.

Regardless of why or when the physical or emotional consequences first appear, they can provide the motivation to now face what we could not face before, and to heal both physically and emotionally. My experience suggests that many of us have the capacity to tolerate emotions that we once needed to keep from awareness.

My patients have shown me the miracle of healing that can occur with awareness. With it, the burden of hypertension and many other illnesses can be transformed into an opportunity for healing. Unfortunately, this opportunity for healing is rarely considered.

Before we heal, we must learn something no one ever taught us: that we have more strength than we realize to face, and heal from, the emotions that we have been hiding. And that we can gain strength from others.

There is a need for healing and a time for healing.

Hidden Emotions in Other Disorders

9

DESPITE CONSIDERABLE RESEARCH, the origin of many highly prevalent physical disorders, such as irritable bowel syndrome, colitis, and chronic fatigue, is still not understood. A mind–body link is suspected in many of them, but research has failed to demonstrate a link to the emotions we feel. Similarly, a mind–body link is suspected but not proven in people with various unexplained physical symptoms such as dizziness, headaches, pain, insomnia, tiredness, poor concentration, and ringing in the ears.

Scientists are now seeking the answer in neurobiology, molecular biology, and genetics, as if emotions were irrelevant. Without doubt they will uncover abnormalities that are involved in some of those conditions and that are targets for drug treatment. However, they will still lack an understanding of why these abnormalities occur and how to cure rather than just treat them.

In medical practice, patients with persisting unexplained physical disorders and symptoms are subjected to test after test, in the hope of finding a cause. However, a cause is rarely uncovered, and they are left with a lifetime of symptoms, pills, and frustration.

The emotions we are aware of usually do not provide an explanation either. If they did, this link would be pretty obvious. The emotions we do not feel can provide an explanation, but physicians rarely consider them.

Ten percent of Americans suffer from insomnia (see G. D. Mellinger, 1985). Most simply assume that it is just the way they are. They are not "good sleepers." Others try to find the reason but usually come up with no answer.

People have tried all sorts of remedies, from warm milk, to a nightcap, to pills, to melatonin, and others. It is no coincidence that the most popular and successful sleeping pills are antianxiety drugs, even though many of the people they help do not claim to be more anxious or under more stress than anyone else. These pills work wonders for many people. Unfortunately, the flip side is that many people cannot sleep without taking them.

Seventeen percent of women and 6 percent of men suffer from migraine headaches (see W. F. Stewart, 1994). Despite advances in treatment, the physical suffering and the number of lost days of work are considerable. Pills help relieve symptoms and prevent attacks, but they do not cure. What is the cause of migraine headaches? Theresa's story in Chapter 5 suggests that hidden emotions may sometimes play an important role.

Twenty to 25 percent of women and 7 to 12 percent of men will develop depression at some point in their life (see the Depression Guideline Panel, 1993). Depression is mediated by, and often blamed on, a chemical imbalance—a reduction in the level of neurotransmitters, such as noradrenaline and serotonin, in the brain. Drugs that increase the levels of these neurotransmitters relieve depression. What is the cause of their reduced levels? Genetics likely explain part of depression but clearly not all of it.

Even though antianxiety pills are used for insomnia and antidepressants are used for various chronic pain disorders, we still rarely consider a link between these disorders and emotions. Again, if the emotions involved were emotions that we were aware of, the link would be obvious. Until we acknowledge that emotions that we do not feel can affect us, the mind–body link will continue to elude us.

The stories that I'll share in this chapter will demonstrate a link between hidden emotions and conditions other than hypertension. They provide tantalizing hints that our hidden emotions are more involved in our health than we realize. Most of these patients also had hypertension, but the effect on blood pressure is not a central part of their story.

Back Pain

Dr. John Sarno, at New York University Medical Center, is the main proponent of a link between hidden emotions and back pain. Influenced by Sarno, many people with back pain that had not responded to medical or surgical treatment experienced dramatic improvement upon realizing that it was related to emotions they were hiding.

Describing his findings in *Healing Back Pain*, Sarno reports that many people who suffered for years experienced relief within hours or days of realizing this link. The rapidity of their response resembles my observations that a healing shift in awareness, by itself, can have rapid effects on blood pressure.

I believe back pain and hypertension share certain similarities. Both are linked to hidden emotions in some people. And, in both conditions, when hidden emotions are contributory, a shift in awareness of them can produce rapid improvement. In either condition, the contribution of both physical and emotional factors must be considered in order to provide the most holistic and appropriate treatment for each individual.

Headaches

An occasional tension headache, just like temporary elevation in blood pressure, can be attributed to day-to-day stress. However, when tension or migraine headaches recur again and again for months or years with no obvious link to stress, their origin is a mystery to us.

My experience suggests that in some people hidden emotions play an important role in the origin of unexplained headaches. Theresa, whose story is presented in Chapter 5, had suffered from migraine headaches for decades. They stopped after a single conversation about the sexual abuse she had suffered in childhood and had hidden away. Deirdre's story also suggests how hidden emotions might explain headaches that are otherwise destined to remain a lifelong mystery.

▸ Deirdre, at sixteen, had had headaches for 12 years. They occurred almost daily, usually midmorning, and lasted for hours. Acetaminophen (Tylenol), aspirin, or ibuprofen (Motrin) used to help but no longer did.

There were no abnormalities on physical examination. She had had an EEG (electroencephalogram), a test that examines brain waves, and it was normal. I referred her to a neurologist, who diagnosed the headaches as migraine, supplying a label but no explanation as to why she was plagued by daily headaches for so many years.

He treated her by proceeding down the long list of medications used for migraine. Imitrex, a recently approved drug for migraine, did not help. A beta blocker did help, but she will have to take it indefinitely. It is not a cure.

Deirdre's headaches were far outside the norm. I talked further with her, hoping to unravel the mystery of why she had them. She had very attentive eyes that conveyed a maturity greater than her years.

I looked for sources of tension. Her father had abandoned the family when she was two, and she had never known him. Her older brother was often sarcastic to her, hardly an uncommon problem. School was school. Her grades were okay. Yes, like many other kids, she had stress, but it did not explain daily headaches for twelve years.

Deirdre did not feel particularly close to her mother. I asked if there was someone else she had felt closer to. Yes, her grandmother. Her grandparents had lived with her from birth, and her grandmother had been a surrogate mother for her when her mother was away for a year after Deirdre's first birthday. Her grandmother died when Deirdre was four or five.

Her grandmother's death and the onset of her headaches occurred at roughly the same age. This could have been merely coincidental, but Deirdre provided another clue. I asked her if she ever suffered nightmares. No, except when she slept with the blanket her grandmother had made for her. Therefore, she had put it away and no longer slept with it.

I suggested that exploring her past with a psychotherapist might be helpful in managing her headaches. I was not surprised that she chose not to. Unaware of the emotions, and in a battle to not feel them, she had no interest in talking about them, no matter how bad her headaches were. She was not yet able to do this.

Someday, when the time is right, I hope she will reconsider. In the meantime, her treatment options are limited to pills. ◄

Deirdre might have to face a lifetime of unexplained headaches and pills to treat them. However, her personal history offers a possible explanation, where CAT (computed axial tomography), MRI (magnetic resonance imaging), and PET (positron emission tomography) scans cannot. She likely blocked extremely painful emotions from awareness, protecting her emotional stability but leaving her with headaches. These emotions include, but are likely not limited to, those related to the death of her surrogate mother when she was four.

Many children lose a grandparent during childhood. For most, it has little effect in the long run. Research studies will never focus on the impact of the death of a grandmother. It was only the details of Deirdre's story, which revealed the early primary caretaker role of her grandmother, that provided the clues of a possible explanation for her headaches.

Raynaud's Phenomenon

► Connie, sixty-four, had borderline hypertension. She had recently suffered a small hemorrhage in her eye. Her borderline hypertension was of questionable relevance to it, but her ophthalmologist suggested that she ought to have the hypertension treated.

For the past eight months she had also suffered episodes of painful constriction of the circulation to her hands and feet, a condition known as Raynaud's phenomenon. This would occur when she was exposed to cold but also inexplicably at many other times.

She had seen a cardiologist, a hematologist, and a rheumatologist, but a multitude of tests did not uncover a cause. She had tried various medications that either had not worked or had bothered her. When she saw me, there were virtually no medications or tests left to try.

Connie's mother had died the previous year, at ninety. At first I did not think that this expected death was relevant. However, Connie told me that she was upset that she had consented to the amputation of her mother's leg, against her mother's specific wishes. Connie had consented because she was told that her mother would die if the gangrenous leg was not amputated. She died anyway, not long afterward. Connie blamed herself for having violated her mother's wishes. I emphasized to her that, under the circumstances, it would have been hard not to give consent.

I assured Connie that constriction of the circulation in her hands and feet was extremely unlikely to ever lead to amputation of her arm or leg. I was surprised at the relief she felt after I said that. She realized she had been worried that her limbs might also have to be amputated someday. It was as if the blood vessel constriction were reproducing in her the risk of amputation that her mother had faced.

With relief both from having aired her feelings about the amputation of her mother's leg and from having been told that her circulatory condition would not lead to amputation, Connie felt much better. She reported that her symptoms lessened by 90 percent, with no medication. Her blood pressure fell to normal, staying in the 120s. A year later, Connie remains well, on no medication. ◄

Heart Arrhythmias

How rapidly our heart beats is controlled by an electrical signaling apparatus, the sinus node, located in the atrium of the heart. A rapid heart rate originating from the sinus node is called a *sinus tachycardia*. It is not caused by abnormality of the heart but by factors such as exertion, fever, anemia, excessive thyroid hormone, or anxiety.

Most people with symptoms of a racing heart have a sinus tachycardia. When a rapid heart rate instead originates outside the sinus node, the problem is usually a conduction abnormality within the heart. Sometimes, especially when the heart rate exceeds 180, it can cause symptoms such as dizziness, shortness of breath, or faintness. At this or even faster rates, it can sometimes be life-threatening.

Its cause can sometimes be traced to a tract of nerves that conducts the abnormal and accelerated signal to the ventricle of the heart. Doctors can prescribe medication or perform a procedure called radiofrequency ablation, in which the abnormal nerve tract is severed to prevent recurrence of the tachycardia.

Without treatment, people with this condition are prone to have recurrent bouts of tachycardia. Nobody can predict when they will recur, or why they recur when they do. Occasionally, they are set off by caffeine, alcohol, or emotional stress. However, their relationship to stress is not a very close one.

▸ Mark, forty-nine, never suffered from heart rhythm disturbances until two months ago. Since then he felt his heart racing many times. An electrocardiogram documented that it was a conduction disturbance rather than a sinus tachycardia.

He avoided caffeine and alcohol, but episodes recurred until he was placed on atenolol (Tenormin), a beta blocker that blocks the effect of adrenaline on the heart.

Mark was under no more stress than usual. When I asked him about the past, he was reluctant to talk. His childhood had been a miserable one. He was dealing with it in his own way, very carefully and rigidly living his life.

I asked if he was feeling any emotions from the past. He acknowledged that those emotions had been bubbling up during the previous two months, coinciding with his heart rhythm disturbance. A year later Mark decided to begin psychotherapy. He stopped his medication and has had no recurrence of the arrhythmia. ◄

Heart rhythm disturbances like Mark's are viewed as a purely medical problem. Mark's story again suggests that the emotions we harbor from long ago may have more of an impact on our physical health than we realize.

Irritable Bowel Syndrome

Douglas Drossman has published very illuminating studies on the highly prevalent problem of irritable bowel syndrome. In an article published in the *Annals of Internal Medicine* in 1990, he reported that women with this disorder or with longstanding unexplained lower abdominal pain were twice as likely as women in a control group to have been sexually abused during childhood.

Very few had discussed the abuse with anyone. I would suspect most dealt with their painful emotions by themselves and blocked them. They likely felt that they had put the abuse behind them and that it had nothing to do with their disorder. Reports such as Dr. Drossman's will help people begin to consider that childhood events can and do affect adult health, long after we have put the emotions related to them behind us.

Insomnia

Many of my patients complain of insomnia. Many of them ask me for an explanation and a cure for it. Needless to say, research has not come up with a good answer, and usually all I can offer is a prescription.

In several patients I have seen insomnia virtually disappear after hidden emotions were uncovered. Theresa was one such patient. The following is the story of another.

> ▶ Margaret developed hypertension only five years ago, when she was fifty-six. It began amidst a number of problems. Her job as an administrator was in jeopardy because her company had been bought out. That same year, her father died at eighty. Margaret also developed insomnia that year, and subsequently her weight climbed 60 pounds.

Margaret clearly had enough stress to upset her at the time, but those events did not seem sufficient to cause persisting hypertension, insomnia, and a 60-pound weight gain. Margaret had never felt that close to her father, anyway.

Margaret also was briefly depressed that year and attributed it to the stirring of grief for her mother, triggered by her father's death. For the first time, she felt like an orphan.

Margaret had been eleven when her mother died. She had been told that her mother had cancer only a week before her mother's death. Margaret told me that at the time she concocted a belief that her mother was not really gone. Eventually she just put her mother out of her mind, for decades, until her father died.

I asked Margaret if she recalled having been close with her mother. Her closeness was evident in the way she spoke. Although talking about her mother might have been upsetting, it was clear that Margaret was cherishing what was a rare opportunity to talk about her.

Margaret never spoke about her mother, not to her father, her daughter, or her boyfriend. Even when she was depressed after her father died and was beginning to finally grieve the loss of her mother, she spoke to no one. Her boyfriend was not interested and suggested that she see a psychiatrist.

All Margaret needed was to be able to talk with someone. But there was nobody. So she did not talk, and instead developed hypertension and insomnia, and gained 60 pounds.

Sharing her story, Margaret felt better. The door to both the grief and the love hidden within was opened in this conversation. Margaret felt both pain and elation, and was both eager and reluctant to pursue her grief. Although she has not yet done the emotional work she needs to do, her insomnia has disappeared. ◄

Margaret would never have guessed that her insomnia was related to hidden emotions about her mother. She also would never have expected a mere conversation to relieve her insomnia. But it did.

I suspect that hidden emotions are related to insomnia in many people. I am describing Margaret's case because a source of hidden emotions became quickly obvious, after which her insomnia quickly disappeared. Treating insomnia is rarely this easy. Nevertheless, in the absence of an explanation or cure for insomnia, I believe it is unwise to overlook the role of hidden emotions.

Panic Disorder

Several years ago, I was involved in a remarkable encounter that steered my attention to hidden emotions.

> ▸ Eric, sixty-three, had come to see me about his blood pressure, not about his episodes of shortness of breath. Two years ago he had begun to experience episodes of shortness of breath that were so disabling and frightening that for two to three hours he could focus on nothing but getting enough air. Sometimes these episodes were accompanied by an ache in his chest. On two or three occasions, he went to a local emergency room, where oxygen and time had relieved his breathlessness. Many tests had been performed to look for coronary disease, asthma, and other conditions. All the tests had yielded normal results.
>
> The symptoms recurred, without warning, every one to two months. He feared for his life and was not reassured by the normal test results. We wondered if anxiety could be causing them, but he insisted he was not anxious about anything other than the attacks.
>
> The recent elevation in his blood pressure readings was only further evidence of his escalating medical problems. He had always had normal readings, but readings of 130–150/100 in the past year had prompted his call to see me.
>
> Since he had symptoms suggestive of panic attacks, I decided to inquire further about the stress in his life.

Eric was tall and slightly overweight and wore dark-framed glasses and a conservative suit. He possessed degrees in law and business and had been a very successful executive. He was currently involved with important business negotiations, but he had been in this position before, and, if anything, relished the challenge. He was well respected for his energy and accomplishments.

He told me he had been very happily married for over thirty years. He had two grown children, both well educated and on a good career track. Eric felt close to both. There had been no recent illness in his family and no major changes in any aspect of his life. Having discovered nothing, I asked him if there was anything he was afraid of.

"I'm afraid of retiring."

"Why?"

"Because I like to look forward to the next thing I'm going to do. You're always judged by your accomplishments. You are what you do."

Eric described how he was at his best when discussing work-related matters. He was not comfortable discussing other things. He was approaching retirement age but had no intention of retiring, as long as it was within his power.

"What about looking back, taking satisfaction from your accomplishments, of which you have so many?"

"I don't like looking back. I prefer looking forward."

I believed that the prospect of retirement was a major concern for him but one that many working adults eventually face. I did not believe it explained his condition.

I wondered why he did not like looking back. A little sheepishly, I asked this high-powered executive about his experiences in the past, particularly as a little boy.

In a very clinical way, he presented the story of his childhood. He was the youngest of eight children. His mother had died when he was three. His father had remarried three years later; his stepmother "didn't like" him, and he was "shipped off" at six to an older sister. Two years later, one of his older brothers was placed in a tuberculosis sanitorium. Although Eric did not recall being sick, he was taken from home and placed in a room with his brother. He remained in the sanitorium for three years, and at eleven, was "shipped off" to another sister. ("I guess the other sister had tired of me.")

Three years later, lying about his age, he joined the military. After his discharge, the GI bill enabled him to pursue the degrees he ultimately obtained and to take charge of his life.

I was struck by the sadness of his story and by how well things had turned out. I could understand why he did not like to look back.

With no explanation for the panic attacks fifty years later, I asked matter-of-factly:

"Do you think your horrible childhood might have anything to do with your current symptoms?"

He looked at me, stunned.

He stuttered: "I . . . don't . . . know. It never occurred to me."

He remained stunned for several minutes. I checked his blood pressure. It was 130/85—normal. We were both surprised.

I saw him two months later. In the interim he had thought a lot about his childhood, for the first time in decades. He even visited the town where he had lived and the sanitorium. He had cried on several occasions, and sometimes he felt as if he were having a conversation with the eight-year-old boy who had lived through that period.

He had delved into the childhood issues much further than I had expected. His blood pressure was again normal. Before he left, I realized he had not mentioned anything about his symptoms.

"By the way, how are the shortness of breath and the chest pain?"

"Oh, I haven't had any."

Three years later, his blood pressure was still normal, and he had had no recurrence of symptoms. ◄

My purpose in relating Eric's story is not to demonstrate an effect on blood pressure. Eric's hypertension was mild and the change in blood pressure was minor and not well documented. The purpose is to note the disappearance of his panic disorder after he became aware of emotions hidden long ago.

Eric's story is consistent with evidence that the root of panic attacks can lie in events that long ago ceased to be consciously distressing. These childhood events could not have been further from Eric's attention than they had been.

Panic disorder does not tend to disappear quickly. I believe Eric's story is a rare one, but one that demonstrates clearly the importance of considering what we have hidden inside us.

Anxiety Disorders

▸ Roberta, twenty-seven, taught children with learning disabilities. She was taking methyldopa (Aldomet) for borderline hypertension. She had suffered two miscarriages and was concerned about the possible effect of her hypertension on future pregnancies. Her blood pressure was normal in my office.

Roberta had suffered from anxiety attacks for the past two to four years, even before the miscarriages. For the past six months the anxiety had been virtually constant, with palpitations, sweats, dizziness, numbness in her left side, and trembling that could last all day.

I asked Roberta what she considered to be the biggest stress in her life. She described teaching. The students just could not learn. This aggravated her and she took this aggravation home, unable to relax even on weekends. Understandably, she felt that this stress was the cause of her problems.

I inquired about Roberta's childhood. Her father had been stern, but even so, her childhood seemed unremarkable.

Although teaching children with learning disabilities is difficult, the unrelenting quality of her anxiety seemed disproportionate. I asked Roberta if she had ever had contact with children like them when she was small. She started crying. Her younger sister had cerebral palsy, and, as a child, Roberta had wanted nothing to do with her. Embarrassed and crying more, she proceeded to recall how happy her sister would be if Roberta merely let her sit with her. Roberta did not let her; she wanted nothing to do with her.

Roberta cried even though she barely knew me. She cried because her sister had been so nice and had asked so little. She cried, feeling her guilt over how little it would have taken to make her sister happy—guilt that she had not felt since she was a child. And this guilt, although hidden, was triggered every day when she saw her students. It is perhaps not a coincidence that she had chosen to work as a special education teacher in the first place, perhaps to undo what she had done as a child.

Roberta's blood pressure remained normal or near normal off medication. Her anxiety and trembling ceased permanently within one or two days. And she began to spend more time with her sister, to make amends for the past. ◄

It would be easy to blame Roberta's anxiety on her job. The clue in this and other cases of the effect of hidden emotions was the disproportion between the stress and the emotional reaction to it. It suggested that her job was a trigger of other emotions, rather than itself being the explanation.

The source of Roberta's anxiety and trembling would not have been detected in a questionnaire about childhood trauma because there had been none. Yet the emotions at their root were disturbing enough for her to have blocked them out. This emphasizes yet again the futility of studying the relationship between emotions and health without getting back to individual people and their stories.

Hidden Depression

Every physician sees patients who are suffering from depression. However, depression that is obvious to both patient and physician is only the tip of the iceberg. In many people, physical symptoms that cannot be explained are the only symptoms of depression. People often do not know that they are depressed.

These are the patients who are the most difficult to diagnose and treat. They complain of aches, pains, fatigue, and other unexplained physical symptoms, not sadness and hopelessness. They might have experienced an unexplained weight loss or weight gain. They might have noticed vague chest pains that tests could not explain.

They are unaware that beneath their physical distress lies depression. They do not feel depressed and insist they are not depressed, even if their life history provides ample reasons for them to be depressed. For them, depression manifests as a physical disorder, and provokes a search for a medical cause and treatment.

Patients with this type of depression consult a physician rather than a psychotherapist. They might feel insulted and angry if the physician suggests that they are depressed and fear he is missing a diagnosis. They often seek another opinion. They seek tests and pain pills, not antidepressants or psychotherapy. They tend to believe the doctor is wrong, and occasionally, the doctor *is* wrong; however, usually he is not. He is exercising good judgment in suggesting the mind–body link.

Treating such patients is not easy. Certainly a physician must consider physical causes and order appropriate diagnostic tests. Even if a patient is depressed, depression can be accompanied by, or complicated by, physical disorders.

However, usually when physical symptoms are not suggestive of any disease process, a medical cause is not found. Doctors can always think of another cause or another test, but at some point doing further tests is unlikely to uncover a diagnosis.

The care of such patients can be very costly and unsatisfying to both patient and physician, with years of tests and pills that do not eliminate the symptoms. Often the symptoms are replaced by new ones, bringing on a new round of tests, pills, and frustration.

The possibility of hidden depression is often hard to see when someone insists he does not feel depressed and does not look depressed. Primary care physicians have been criticized for failure to diagnose depression, but, in fairness, depression often is not obvious when it manifests as physical rather than emotional distress.

When we consider the possibility that the source of intractible physical symptoms lies in hidden depression, the door is open to psychotherapy and/or antidepressant drugs. Treating the depression can finally relieve the symptoms and bring an end to the otherwise endless cycle of feeling sick and seeking doctors. Thus, even when a person with a history of longstanding unexplained physical symptoms does not feel depressed, physicians and family members should not overlook the possibility of a hidden depression.

IN THE CASE HISTORIES IN THIS CHAPTER, patients came to me without intending to address emotional issues. Their stories indicate that a healing shift in awareness of hidden emotions can follow the simple telling and sharing of our inner secrets, the telling of our story for the first time. Some of these encounters were truly remarkable ones, marked by dramatic and rapid improvement. Some may have been simply lucky cases. However, most appear to have been more than that.

For some reason, in these case histories the fit between patient and me, the ease of communication, the timing, and other factors were just right. Perhaps it was the inquiry by a physician rather than a psychotherapist. Perhaps some patients were a hair away from awareness, separated only by the nudge needed to recognize the role of emotions they had hidden from themselves. Perhaps through my experience I have learned to ask the right questions. Perhaps it was because I simply listened and respected their distress without rushing to abort it. Most important, maybe I was the only person they encountered who inquired about their past and about things that were not bothering them.

In 1993, Dale Matthews, in an article in the *Annals of Internal Medicine*, and William Zinn, in an article in the *Archives of Internal Medicine*, described the importance of an empathetic relationship between doctor and patient. Defining empathy as the sharing, with a sense of connectedness, of another person's experience, they describe how this relationship allows patients ventilation of their emotional distress and contributes to a sense of relief. I would add to their description the relief provided by the sharing of emotions that have been hidden, even for decades.

I do not mean to suggest that dramatic improvement will always follow the mere telling of a story. Obviously it will not. However, occasionally it can, particularly if a person gains awareness of previously hidden emotions. Even without dramatic improvement, understanding the basis of the symptoms or disorder can also point the way toward a healing path.

THE EXPLANATIONS FOR THE DISORDERS discussed in this chapter are rarely found in the emotions people feel and report. My observations suggest instead that they may be found in hidden emotions. This is the heart of the challenge of mind–body medicine: to recognize the link between physical symptoms and emotions when there is no emotional distress to lead our way to it.

There is a disturbing trend that dominates medicine and psychiatry today. More and more conditions are being studied as if they bear no link to emotions. Research has led to successful drug treatment, although the drugs must be taken indefinitely because they do not cure.

We can treat these ailments medically, but to fully understand them and possibly cure them we must begin to look at the role of hidden emotions.

PART

3

Healing

Are Hidden Emotions Causing Your Hypertension?

10

H IDDEN EMOTIONS, or emotions of any kind, are certainly not the only cause of hypertension. In many people genetics or obesity or other factors are largely at its root, and hidden emotions are not.

I believe that hidden emotions contribute to hypertension in roughly a quarter to half of people with hypertension. How then can you tell if your hypertension is related to hidden emotions? My experience indicates that there are many helpful clues.

During years of one-on-one contact with patients I began to notice patterns that suggested when hidden emotions were relevant and when they were not. Among them are the pattern and severity of your hypertension, the symptoms associated with it, and the personal history that you bring along with you. I will explain all of these and what they mean to you.

Clues to the Role of Hidden Emotions in Hypertension
- ▸ The pattern of your hypertension
- ▸ The severity of your hypertension
- ▸ Hypertension accompanied by other disorders of unknown origin
- ▸ Your personal history

The Pattern of Your Hypertension

Hypertension research has paid remarkably little attention to what the pattern of a person's hypertension tells us about its cause.

Certain patterns stand out in suggesting that something other than genetic essential hypertension is going on. They beg for an explanation—an explanation that hidden emotions can provide.

Clues Provided by the Pattern of Your Hypertension
- Episodic hypertension unrelated to obvious stress
- Abrupt and unexplained onset of hypertension
- Hypertension in someone with no risk factors for hypertension
- Uncontrollable hypertension
- Hypertension beginning at a young age

Episodic Hypertension Unrelated to Obvious Stress
Even if we do not have hypertension, it is normal for our blood pressure to rise, sometimes considerably, with excitement, fear, or anger. In many people blood pressure can soar while it is being measured. These increases bear an obvious relationship to the circumstances in which they occur.

However, as discussed in Chapter 7, some people experience marked blood pressure elevation seemingly out of nowhere, with no obvious emotional cause. One moment their blood pressure is fine and the next moment it is high, remaining elevated for minutes, hours, or longer. With this elevation, some feel sick. Others do not.

If your blood pressure follows this pattern, an origin in hidden emotions is extremely likely. Even if you are feeling no emotional distress and no source of stress is immediately apparent to you, there is likely to be emotion inside that begs to be heard. If you can acknowledge and address it, the hypertension can ease, or even be cured. Even if you cannot do so, or choose not to, recognizing the origin of the hypertension in hidden emotions can be helpful in guiding selection of medications to control it, as discussed in Chapters 7 and 13.

Abrupt and Unexplained Onset of Hypertension
Essential hypertension can be expected to develop gradually, at first with readings that fluctuate above and below the upper limit

of normal. Eventually most readings are above normal, and hypertension is diagnosed and treatment is considered.

In contrast, if your blood pressure has always been normal and without explanation rises substantially, for example, from 120/80 to 170/100, and remains elevated, your physician will strongly suspect that something other than genetic essential hypertension is going on. He is likely to embark on a search for unusual and curable causes of hypertension such as narrowing of an artery to a kidney (particularly in smokers); excessive production of hormones such as aldosterone, cortisol, or adrenaline; or other causes. Occasionally he will find a cause. Usually he will not.

There should be a reason for sudden-onset hypertension. Genetics cannot explain it. If you just found out that you were about to be laid off from your job, it makes sense, although even in this circumstance, the blood pressure elevation will usually be temporary and relatively mild: 10 or 20 millimeters, not 50. If you recently gained 40 pounds, an increase in blood pressure makes sense, although I would also suspect that emotions are involved in a rapid weight gain of that magnitude. I would also consider the possibility that anxiety following a single high reading provoked high readings during subsequent measurements. Monitoring your blood pressure away from your physician's office can help assess this possibility.

Even when an obvious cause is not apparent, it is tempting to ascribe blame to a recent minor stressful event, such as a work deadline or a daughter's obnoxious new boyfriend. Such events can also raise your blood pressure a bit but cannot explain a marked and sustained elevation.

Investigation for uncommon medical causes should not be overlooked in a rush to find an emotional basis. Unfortunately, once the tests come back negative, patients and physicians are resigned to the diagnosis of essential hypertension and lifelong drug treatment. I believe, however, that the same logic that dictated the search for a medical cause should also provoke a search for an emotional basis. A search for hidden emotions might be the only way left to make sense of your hypertension. An opportunity is missed if this is not considered and care is limited to lifelong drug therapy.

Hypertension in Someone with No Risk Factors for Hypertension

If you have no family history of hypertension, are young and thin, and do not have an obvious burden of severe current stress, it will seem to you and your physician that you shouldn't have hypertension. I am careful to make sure that patients in this category truly have hypertension and not white coat hypertension, as discussed in Chapter 2. However, if you truly have more than minimal hypertension, consideration of hidden emotions might be the only way to make sense of it.

Uncontrollable Hypertension

In some people, despite the excellent drugs available, hypertension cannot be brought under control. Joel Menard, in a review published in the *American Journal of Hypertension* in 1992, found that in several major studies treatment failed to lower blood pressure to normal in as many as a third of people with hypertension. Using the wrong medication or dose is often the problem. Sometimes the problem is the failure to take the medication.

However, in some people, like Martha in Chapter 5, the blood pressure remains elevated no matter what medication is prescribed. A search for uncommon medical causes is warranted but usually nothing is found. Medical research cannot explain this resistance to treatment, especially given the long list of excellent drugs available. In my experience, in most patients with truly uncontrollable hypertension, a basis in hidden emotions is very likely. Considering this possibility might be the only way to make sense of the hypertension and to better control it.

Hypertension Beginning at a Young Age

It is uncommon for sustained hypertension to appear in a teenager. Unfortunately, in most, after the necessary tests are done, a cause is not identified. I believe hidden emotions can provide an explanation in many.

The Severity of Your Hypertension

According to the recent report of the Joint National Committee on Detection, Evaluation and Treatment of High Blood Pressure (see V. A. Pogue, 1996), 21 percent of people with hypertension have mild hypertension, 35 percent have moderate hypertension, and 44 percent have severe hypertension. The risk of complications increases with the severity of the hypertension. I believe the likelihood that hidden emotions are contributory increases as well.

Borderline Hypertension

If you have borderline hypertension (blood pressure in the 130s or 140s/80s or 90s), studies indicate a 50 percent likelihood that you will never develop sustained hypertension, as reviewed by Stevo Julius in 1971. If the elevation is a result of temporary stress, it will usually subside on its own. Sometimes, exercising, losing weight, or reducing your salt intake is all you need to do. It is also possible that you are simply reacting to the blood pressure measurement itself, as discussed in Chapter 2.

With borderline hypertension there is a considerable overlap between who has hypertension and who does not. It is wrong to believe that if your blood pressure is 142/92, you differ greatly from someone with a blood pressure of 138/88. Similarly, the risk of cardiovascular complications is minimally different. If you are in this category, I would not rush to explore hidden emotions to explain it.

Mild Hypertension

Mild hypertension is usually easy to control with nondrug measures or with a pill or two a day. The mild blood pressure elevation often can be explained by factors such as genetics, weight, and day-to-day stress. I would not look for a basis in hidden emotions if your hypertension disappears with a reduction in salt intake or a little exercise. Even if your hypertension requires a pill or two a day, if it is easily controlled and not associated with physical or emotional symptoms, it may have little to do with hidden emotions. You would also have little motivation to pursue such a cause.

On the other hand, if you are thin and have no conspicuous stress, if no one in your family had hypertension, and the above measures do not normalize your blood pressure, the hypertension might be more of a mystery to you. If you wonder why you have it, you might find the explanation in hidden emotions. The pattern of your hypertension, the symptoms associated with it, and your personal history provide further clues of whether hidden emotions are involved.

Moderate to Severe Hypertension
If you are in this group, no matter what its cause, your hypertension is unlikely to disappear on its own and medication is likely to be required, probably for the rest of your life. Ways to find the right drug or drugs are discussed in Chapter 13.

The more severe your hypertension, the more likely your doctor will want to perform tests to search for an uncommon medical cause. Gunnar Anderson, in a study published in 1994, found a cause in roughly 10 percent of people whose diastolic blood pressure was above 110. However, in 90 percent he could not find a cause.

You would think that if the emotional distress we are aware of caused hypertension, it would be most obvious in those with severe hypertension. Yet even in this group, that link is not apparent. In my own research as well, as reported in the *Journal of Psychosomatic Research* in 1998, hypertension was not related to the anger and anxiety people reported, even among those with severe hypertension. My experience indicates instead that emotions that we do not feel can make sense of hypertension in many people in this group, particularly in those with the most severe hypertension.

Hypertension Accompanied by Other Disorders of Unknown Origin

There are many disorders, such as migraine, asthma, insomnia, nightmares, various chronic pain syndromes, unexplained weight gain, and colitis, whose origin, like that of hypertension, is not well understood. Genetic predisposition plays a role in some but cannot fully explain these disorders. Emotions are suspected of playing a role, but, again, the emotions we are aware of have not provided an explanation.

The origin of these disorders might also lie in hidden emotions. And when they accompany hypertension, I tend to suspect more strongly that hidden emotions are contributory to both conditions. If you have conditions such as these in addition to your hypertension, hidden emotions might be playing a role even if you are certain they are not. The cases in Chapter 9 indicate how considering them can be important in restoring your health.

Your Personal History

▸ Clara, sixty-one, had hypertension for only one year. She was under a lot of stress and came to see me to determine whether or not emotional distress was causing her hypertension.

At her doctor's office, Clara's blood pressure had been about 150–155/95–100 over the past few months, even though she was taking losartan (Cozaar), an angiotensin II antagonist (see Chapter 13). Her blood pressure was 150/95 in my office. She was not overweight. Her father, who had died at eight-six, had had mild hypertension.

Her father had died two years earlier. Her mother, who was eight-five and dependent on her, was living with her and her husband. Her mother was very demanding of her time. Clara felt trapped. She was tense and increasingly angry, realizing the extent to which her mother, now and in the past, had controlled her life. And, no matter how much she did for her mother, Clara felt guilty. She wasn't doing enough.

Clara suspected that the recent onset of her hypertension was related to this stress. She clearly was feeling a lot of emotional distress and seemed to be in touch with an array of appropriate but troubling emotions. Her awareness of those emotions did not fit the mind–body link that I have come to expect. I asked her if she ever checked her blood pressure at home. She said she did but that her monitor was inaccurate; the readings were normal. I checked her monitor. It was accurate. Now off medication, her blood pressure has remained normal. ◄

Clara had come to me to determine whether or not emotions were driving her hypertension. She did not consider a third possibility, that she did not have hypertension. Her awareness of her feelings was the clue that suggested that her blood pressure might be normal outside of the doctor's office.

Clara is dealing with her distressing emotions with the help of a psychotherapist. I expect that her discomfort and her attention to those emotions will lead her to a successful resolution of the conflicts facing her.

IT IS USUALLY EASY to identify people like Clara who are in touch with their distressful emotions. They tell me they are feeling distressed. People who conceal their emotions cannot tell me they are hiding distressful emotions. However, there are many clues that indicate they are doing so. You might recognize them in yourself or in someone close to you.

Clues to a Burden of Hidden Emotions
- Emotional trauma that you think is behind you
- Not feeling unwanted emotions (see Chapter 6)
- A history suggestive of emotional isolation
- Childhood abuse or severe family dysfunction
- Certainty that hidden emotions do not affect you

Emotional Trauma That You Think Is Behind You
Patients who have hypertension, particularly severe hypertension, and a history of severe emotional trauma, regularly claim that

they have put it behind them and feel no lingering effects. When they say this, it is usually crystal clear to me that they have blocked emotions and that the threat of awareness of those emotions might be relevant to the hypertension.

They might have felt distress at the time of the trauma and therefore believe they have dealt with those emotions. Even so— and this is key—if they insist that the trauma has left no lingering emotion at all, it is likely that there are hidden layers of emotion that could be affecting their blood pressure.

On the other hand, when a patient can tell me that he has dealt with trauma and recovered but can still get teary when he recalls the past, or acknowledge that he will never completely get over it, he is telling me that he is aware of these emotions. I have found hypertension to be much less common in trauma survivors who have this awareness.

Usually it is easy to tell who is, and who is not, aware of those emotions. Ironically, the tendency has always been to implicate painful emotions as a cause of illness only in the people who feel them. My experience suggests the opposite, that it is the emotions we are not aware of that are more likely to lead to hypertension and other physical disorders.

Not Feeling Unwanted Emotions

If you tend to be emotionally involved in your relationships and in general feel distress commensurate with the situations you face, I would be inclined to believe that your hypertension is not principally driven by emotions. If you are under stress and feel tense, I would suspect emotions are not driving your hypertension beyond temporary elevation. If, on the other hand, you tend to stay at a very even keel, as I've discussed in Chapter 6, emotions you do not feel are more likely to be a factor in your hypertension.

If much of your emotional distress is unfelt, you will probably find it hard to believe that emotions could be relevant to your hypertension, even if it is evident to others that you are holding in a lot of emotion. If you are remarkably calm in the face of enormous stress that most people think should be bothering you, if you are seen as an incredibly nice guy, if you try to please everyone and let nothing bother you, and you have considerable hypertension, it might be emotion-based, even though you feel calm.

A History Suggestive of Emotional Isolation

If you enjoyed mutual closeness and respect with a parent or anyone during your childhood, you likely tend to connect with, and confide in, those around you as an adult. If you tend not to connect with and confide in the people in your life, and you feel you don't need anyone, it is likely that you grew up without these experiences. The more stress you have faced in your life, the more likely you will pay a price for handling stress in this isolated way.

Childhood Abuse or Severe Family Dysfunction

I encounter many people who have been abused in one way or another during childhood and are aware that it affected them into adulthood. It is more striking to me when patients tell me the abuse they suffered did not affect them, no matter how severe it was. Some had sufficient emotional resources during childhood to lessen the impact of the abuse on them, and the mildness of the lingering impact makes sense. Others did not, and their insistence that this abuse had no lingering effect suggests hidden effects that may be relevant to their hypertension.

Certainty That Hidden Emotions Do Not Affect You

When I am talking with a patient, I often cannot state with certainty that hidden emotions are contributing to his or her hypertension, even if clues strongly suggest that they are. The fact that someone endured trauma in the past does not prove it is necessarily related to the hypertension. As I described in Chapter 5, when I suggested to Theresa that the severe sexual abuse she had put behind her might be relevant to her hypertension and migraine headaches, I could not be certain about that link until after the improvement in those conditions was evident.

When I offer such an explanation, some patients are willing to consider the possibility that their past is affecting them. Others are not. They are certain that their past does not affect them.

Since we do not and cannot know the extent of our hidden emotions, this certainty is paradoxically a clue that hidden emotions are a considerable threat.

THERE ARE MANY CLUES that can indicate whether hidden emotions are relevant to your hypertension. Was your hypertension gradual in onset or sudden? Is it mild or severe? Is your hypertension episodic? Does it respond to medication?

Do you suffer from other physical or emotional conditions of unknown origin? Have you suffered abuse or trauma in the past? Do you feel affected by it or not?

Do you live your life on a very even keel? Are you relatively immune to both the upsets and the closeness that you see in other people's lives?

The answers to these questions provide clues that indicate whether you are defending yourself from a lot of emotion. If you are, paying attention to those emotions can help you in managing your hypertension.

CHAPTER 11

Healing Hypertension by Honoring Our Emotions

I F I HAD TO SINGLE OUT any aspect crucial to healing emotion-linked hypertension, it would be the realization that we harbor emotions that we don't feel and that they can affect us physically. It has been remarkable to me to see the impact of this shift in awareness.

This shift can come about quickly, and by itself can sometimes alleviate hypertension and other physical problems. We move toward wholeness within ourselves as we integrate parts that we have cut off. This does not mean that all of our problems are solved overnight, nor does it mean that there will not be setbacks. Emotional healing does not occur that rapidly. However, the awareness we gain always creates some change that cannot be taken away, and it finally opens the door to emotional healing.

The shift lies in respecting our emotions rather than ignoring them. It means trusting the healing effect of paying attention to them, even if doing so leads to feeling considerable distress.

The emotions we are hiding come in many guises. We might be convinced we do not harbor them, or we might suspect we do. They might be related to a specific event, or to circumstances that existed for years or decades. They might be related to recent events or to events from long ago. They might be related to abuse or trauma from the past, or might instead reflect a way of being in which we learned without knowing it to routinely hide emotions from ourselves.

My experience tells me over and over that when emotions are knocking at the door of awareness, the person who continues to knowingly or unknowingly guard against recognizing them and is convinced that he or she is not affected by them is more likely to develop hypertension and other physical problems. Fortunately, we retain that option of awareness when we feel we are ready.

Emotions We Don't Know We're Avoiding

We were born with the ability to block out emotions without even knowing we are doing so. We used this ability when we were confronted with more than we were able to handle emotionally. We might have blocked out the pain of emotional trauma or the more routine distress that we could not face growing up emotionally alone. Blocking it out protected us and our ability to function well. Unknowingly we continue to fight to keep emotions from awareness, even when we no longer need to do this.

Martha's and Theresa's stories, presented in Chapter 5, show vividly how emotions related to traumatic events can underlie hypertension beginning even decades later and how gaining awareness of those emotions can relieve hypertension. Martha's hypertension became controllable only when she finally became aware of hidden emotions concerning a decades-old trauma of rape. Finally feeling them was the only way to escape the havoc of battling to avoid them. She was able to face now what she could not have faced before, even though until the moment they surfaced she had no idea that hidden emotions were affecting her.

Theresa's hypertension, headaches, and insomnia improved quickly once she acknowledged the lingering impact of abuse she thought she had put behind her long ago. For the first time in her life, she is able to talk about that abuse, rather than bearing it alone and hiding it as she did as a child. However, her trauma was extensive and true emotional healing will take much longer.

The Pain of Children Losing Parents

The emotional effects in adulthood of abuse incurred in childhood has received considerable attention. The potential physical effects have received less attention. The physical effects of another childhood trauma, the death of a parent, have also received little attention. I have spoken with many patients who endured such a loss. Jimmy, whose story is told in Chapter 6, is one such example. His approach to life and his consequent hypertension can be traced back to events surrounding his mother's death. Margaret's story in Chapter 9 suggests a link between the ungrieved loss of a parent and insomnia. Deirdre's story in Chapter 9 suggests a link to migraine headaches. The following two cases illustrate two paths taken by people who hid emotions concerning the premature loss of a parent.

▶ Jill's blood pressure had always been 110/70, very normal. However, while seeing her doctor because of pain in her knee, she told him she had been having a mild headache for two days. He found her blood pressure to be extremely elevated, at 200/140. She was referred to me and I admitted her into the hospital and lowered her blood pressure with medication.

The obvious question was, Why did she suddenly have severe hypertension? It begged for an explanation. A battery of tests was unrevealing. There was no recent stress that could make sense of it either. However, her past history offered clues.

The first clue was that Jill's mother had died suddenly at fifty-one after a stroke, when Jill was nineteen. At that young age, it was not unlikely that Jill hid a lot of the pain.

Jill was now a month away from turning fifty-one, the same age her mother had been when she died. The coincidence of her hypertensive crisis occurring the year she reached her mother's age is not a rare one, as dormant emotions are stirred up in what has come to be called an "anniversary phenomenon."

Other clues that hidden emotions concerning her mother might be involved were easy to find. Although Jill told me she had been very close with her mother, she remembered grieving for only a few days and invariably forgot about the anniversary of her death, year after year.

Jill had become very close to her mother-in-law and felt more like a daughter to her than a daughter-in-law. On the day Jill was admitted to the hospital with the hypertensive crisis, her mother-in-law was due to undergo surgery at the same hospital in which Jill's mother had died.

One final clue: Jill had felt shaken a few days before when her sister told her for the first time that she now looked just like her mother.

After we talked, Jill acknowledged the possibility of a link between her severe hypertension and emotions locked away long ago. She was a little tearful during our discussion, indicating that the door to those emotions was not shut tight. However, she was not yet ready to deal with those emotions and has not yet sought to do so. She continues to take medication for her hypertension. ◄

From a medical standpoint, Jill's hypertension was a total mystery. However, with all the clues before us, she could understand that it might be linked to her long-hidden emotions. Her blood pressure was the alarm that deep within those emotions were stirring. Unlike Theresa, Jill did not choose to face those emotions. She is not suffering emotional distress and does not feel sufficiently ill to overcome her hidden decades-old fear of facing them. However, an alternative to lifelong medication is available to her, when she is ready.

MANY PEOPLE WHO LOST A PARENT during their childhood or adolescence and believe they put it behind them long ago do not realize that it can be affecting them decades later. In my experience, those who develop hypertension are likely to tell me that they just moved on. They are usually certain that their parent's death had little lingering effect on them and has nothing to do with their hypertension. Those who do not develop hypertension are much more likely to tell me what a devastating loss their parent's death was.

Sometimes the grief is truly inaccessible to awareness. With it, much of the love for that parent also remains inaccessible. When we cut ourselves off from our grief, we also cut off our love for one of the towering figures in our lives. However, even decades later, the child who hasn't grieved might be just a conversation away from awareness and from that love, as I learned from Nancy's story.

▶ When Nancy, now fifty-six, was eleven years old, her mother died of kidney failure caused by severe hypertension. She told me she did not grieve or communicate her emotions to anyone at the time of her mother's death. She had been an only child and her father did not discuss feelings. Left alone with her grief, at eleven, she needed to block her grief and did so. She also blocked the love and closeness she had shared with her mother.

Years later, in her first year of college, her roommates were talking about their mothers and asked Nancy about hers. Nancy began to cry. As she put it, she "broke down." Actually, it was not a breakdown. It was a healing awareness of painful emotions. The tears she was trying to avoid were the healing tears that she needed. She then grieved and for ten years could not speak about her mother without crying.

She no longer cries. She fully feels her love for her mother and her mother's love for her. She can sense her mother's presence with her whenever she wants.

Nancy has a strong genetic predisposition for hypertension and is also overweight at five-six and 185 pounds. Not surprisingly, she has hypertension, but it is very easily controlled with a diuretic—a water pill—taken once a day. Her hypertension is not emotion-driven. ◀

Nancy could not have tolerated feeling the brunt of her grief when she was eleven and alone. Although she was unaware that it was hidden within and although she was not consciously seeking to feel it, her grief poured out as soon as the opportunity arose. It took ten years to empty out the pain, but it enabled her to reconnect with the love she had shared with her mother.

I am amazed at how few of my patients who lost a parent during childhood can tell me that someone was there with them to support them during their grief. Usually the surviving parent, particularly when the death was sudden, was engrossed in his or her own grief, and in merely surviving, emotionally and financially.

Any attention given to surviving children likely consisted of trying to divert them from their grief rather than honoring their grieving process. The pain of their devastating loss was handled alone, and they had to hide much of the emotion. Those children who had the opportunity to share their grief with a parent, or who were engulfed by a grandparent or a close extended family or community, are the lucky exceptions.

Many people who were orphaned during childhood go through life without ever feeling the grief or the love hidden inside. Ironically, they might be as close as a conversation away from a shift in awareness of those emotions. Unfortunately, that conversation may never happen. It is a conversation that never occurs to them to seek, and one that no one initiates. I hope that this book might serve as that conversation.

The Hazards of Hiding Our Emotions Day After Day

► Marian, a vivacious forty-nine-year-old, first experienced a severe headache eight months before seeing me. It was so severe that she was hospitalized, but tests did not yield any diagnosis. The headache eased over several days and finally disappeared.

Four months later, Marian's blood pressure was found to be markedly elevated. Subsequently it was normal at times and very elevated at others. As is often the case, her blood pressure elevation bore no relationship to any ongoing stress or emotion. If anything, her life was on a more even keel than it had been in years.

Marian's doctor prescribed enalapril (Vasotec), an ACE (angiotensin-converting enzyme) inhibitor, but stopped it because it caused a persistent cough. Her blood pressure climbed back up to 180/100. Atenolol (Tenormin), a beta blocker, caused shortness of breath. Marian's blood pressure again rose to 180/105, accompanied by a severe headache. She was then placed on amlodipine (Norvasc), a calcium channel blocker, which lowered her blood pressure.

The lability of Marian's blood pressure, unrelated to any current stress, strongly suggested to me that emotions below the surface were involved. Marian had gained sixty pounds during the previous eighteen months, suggesting either a hormonal or emotional basis for her condition. Tests had not revealed a hormonal cause.

She told me that she grew up with two loving parents and a brother and sister, and was still close to all of them. There had been no alcoholism, no abuse, no neglect.

Marian was a divorcée and had opened a small business that was doing well. She had two grown children.

Marian had sought the divorce because of physical abuse. She had considered her husband the love of her life. However, he was jealous and verbally abusive, and on three occasions nearly strangled her in anger. On one of those occasions she lost consciousness, yet stayed with him for more than a year afterward.

Marian felt she had handled this better than most and had not fallen apart, and that her condition was not related to emotions. The previous doctor had suggested that her illness was in her head and she was furious at him. Yet she acknowledged to me that she had been losing her temper frequently and was not herself. Two years ago she had been a totally different person.

She had also been depressed two years ago, for the better part of a year. She didn't know why. Luckily, the depression lifted by itself. When it did, her headaches and hypertension began.

Marian's hypertension, headaches, weight gain, personality change, previous depression, and history of physical abuse all suggested an emotional basis. Yet she insisted she was one of the most together people she knew. She handled her problems and was always there for everyone.

I asked her who took care of her. She said no one. She took care of herself. When things had been at their worst, she had remained so upbeat that everyone had called her a "Pollyanna," exactly the pattern I have come to associate with hypertension.

I asked her: "You take care of your problems. Do you take care of yourself, of your emotions about what you've been through?"

She paused and then began to cry. She had not allowed herself to heal from the events she had endured. She had shared her problems, but had not felt or shared her deep-felt emotions. Even after gaining sixty pounds, after a depression, after developing headaches and hypertension, she had still been unable to see that there was any emotional storm inside her, any explanation for the downward spiral in her inner life.

I took Marian off all medication and her blood pressure has remained normal. She cried the first few days after our discussion. Then she became angry over the unfairness she perceived in her relationships. Even with this anger, her blood pressure remained very normal, as low as 114/74.

She lost her constant desire for food and within four months lost thirty-five pounds. Her headaches were gone and she felt better.

Feeling on top of the world, Marion stopped doing the work of emotional healing, of facing the painful emotions about her life and how she was living it. Nine months later her symptoms returned briefly. Again she quickly recognized the mind–body link and the symptoms disappeared. Even with the quick relief, Marian is not yet committed to engaging the painful task of healing. A healing path is available, but only if she chooses it. ◄

Marian's health changed once she had shifted awareness and realized how she had been ignoring her emotions. Having always been upbeat and a problem solver, she had seen herself as the last person in whom emotional pain would be a cause of hypertension and headaches.

Her course is also interesting with respect to her weight loss. I encourage many patients to change their diets and lose weight. Some do. Many don't. Ironically, Marian's weight loss required not one iota of encouragement from me. We had not even discussed losing weight.

Marian's course also illustrates how easy it is to abandon a healing path when we feel good. It explains why it takes a big jolt to begin the work of emotional healing. With anything less, we usually don't choose the painful path of the healing process.

Our Biggest Barrier: We Don't Realize
Even if we are unaware of the emotions we hid long ago, they have not been erased from our brain. As reviewed by Rhawn

Joseph and by Elliott Ross, considerable evidence indicates that our painful emotions are stored in the brain's right hemisphere, tucked away from our conscious left brain. In this way, painful emotions can remain a secret of the right brain. We are unaware of them and can swear we do not feel or even harbor them, as long as they are blocked from communication to the left brain. Like Leonard, in Chapter 5, we can insist we escaped unscathed from trauma as severe as the sudden death of a child. However, these emotions remain and can affect us, even decades later.

It would be nice if when they affected us they unambiguously announced themselves. Unfortunately, usually they do not. Unlike the emotions we feel and are aware of, these emotions can affect us physically, without our consciously feeling any emotional distress. This is why the people most likely to have an emotional basis for their hypertension or other unexplained physical condition are least likely to be aware of it or to have sought to do anything about it. They may end up going from doctor to doctor and never imagine that their ailment is related to emotions, even if the explanation is suggested. Neither patient nor physician sees the opportunity for healing.

Our biggest barrier to healing is simply that it has never occurred to us that we are affected by emotions we are not feeling. It is both simple and profound to change that. If you are reading this book, you have the option right now to realize this.

When you look back at what happened to you in the past, especially during your childhood, does it make sense to you that you hid from yourself much of the terror, sadness, or helplessness that could have overwhelmed you at the time? And that hiding them was exactly the right thing to do to protect yourself? And does it make sense that if you hid them, as ample evidence has demonstrated, those emotions persist inside and could be affecting you? And does it make sense that you are now better able to face them and have the choice to do so, to begin a healing process?

Many of us continue to hide our emotions long after our need to do so has waned. The problem usually is not our inability to handle what we decide to allow into awareness. The problem is that we can handle much more than we allow, especially with the right support.

The Rapid Effect of a Shift in Awareness

The effects on physical health of recognizing hidden emotions is sometimes dramatic and rapid, as seen in Martha's and Theresa's stories. Eric and Roberta, whose stories were presented in Chapter 9, and Marian and others similarly benefited almost immediately. This rapid effect resembles very closely the dramatic improvement that John Sarno has noted in some people with back pain once they realize they are hiding emotions from themselves.

It seems unbelievable, but it can follow the mere telling of the story we have told no one for decades. For some of us, it can come after realizing for the first time that hidden emotions can affect us. It can even come from the reading of a book, if awareness is triggered.

With this shift in awareness, the door is then open to further steps to healing. Many resources can help nurture that process, as discussed in the next chapter.

We Have a Choice of Awareness

Should all people in whom hidden emotions are contributing to hypertension be urged to acknowledge and feel them? Or are there some who risk trouble if they seek to recognize and feel that which they locked away from awareness? Sometimes it is difficult to know. Some people can quickly grasp the possible link of their hypertension or other ailment to hidden emotions and are clearly ready to choose a healing pathway. Others cannot. Some may be able to consider this link only months or years later, often motivated by continuing illness. And some never do.

I feel it is important that I describe to patients the possible link to hidden emotions, providing them with a choice of whether to address that link. It is also important that I respect their choice. If the patient is a survivor of unusually severe and brutal trauma, or is too unsettled in her current life, or lacking in emotional support, to engage old pain, her refusal to consider this link is an important indicator that it may be wise to leave well enough alone.

Fortunately, people who should not confront long-hidden emotions generally don't choose to do so. They are more likely to insist that they already dealt with those emotions or that their hypertension, although unexplained, has nothing to do with emotions. The mere suggestion that they harbor these emotions will not cause them to fall apart. If it is unsafe, they are unlikely to pursue this course.

We are lucky in that a shift in awareness is not a choice that we ponder and then decide about. It is instead a choice that seems to happen to us, if we are open to it. The shift in awareness, if it occurs, is itself important evidence that we are ready to confront these hidden emotions. We are unlikely to choose to suddenly unblock emotions that we have been able to shut out for decades unless we are ready to face them. Our instinctual decision is unlikely to present us with more than we are prepared to face.

Emotions That Deep Down We Know We Are Avoiding

The paradigm for healthy handling of our distressful emotions is to face them, preferably in an atmosphere of support and connectedness, and then move on. However, the reality is quite different. Many of us choose to avoid them.

We may be afraid that if we yield control and allow ourselves to feel difficult emotions, we will never be able to shut the door on them; we may fall apart unless we keep that door shut. Avoiding them, we begin to believe that we will never need to deal with them, and we often succeed in forgetting about them. Unfortunately, if we do not pause to acknowledge and even embrace them, these emotions will persist and are likely to affect us.

The fear of falling apart is a major barrier to the healing process. Many people would be surprised to know that they can experience the emotions that are knocking on the door of their awareness without falling apart. Realizing this can be very empowering in breaking the cycle of avoiding emotion and suffering physical illness as a result.

In people who are truly unaware of the emotions triggering their hypertension, the shift needed is one of awareness. However, in people who deep down know they are avoiding emotions, the shift needed is one of choosing to face them, instead of continuing to avoid them no matter what the price. If you are in this category, you have the option to trust yourself, to get the right support, and to stop hiding.

Being Afraid of Falling Apart

▶ When Marj saw me, her blood pressure was 150/90. She had been diagnosed with hypertension a year and a half before and was on a diuretic. She was afraid she needed more medication.

Marj, forty-nine, slim and attractive, with long dark hair, seemed friendly but nervous. She lived alone, enjoyed her work as a public relations consultant, and had many friends.

She had left her husband a year and a half earlier, after an unhappy marriage of twenty-five years. Since then she had been seeing, on an irregular basis, a man who was not seeking a long-term relationship with her. When he stopped seeing her, she became very upset, feeling alone and depressed. She was trying to ignore her distress, but was on the verge of tears even at work, where the tough facade she had always presented was breaking down. She told me she could not control her feelings anymore and feared she was falling apart.

Marj had known from the start that the relationship, one of convenience, was going nowhere. The depth of her emotional reaction seemed disproportionate, suggesting that deeper blocked-off emotions, rather than the breakup itself, were responsible for the severity of her distress.

Her marriage had always been an unhappy one. She had done as her husband had wanted, over time growing more and more unhappy. She had wanted children but he said no. Marj told me that once she finally separated, she quickly bounced back with the help of the new relationship. She had seemingly been very resilient.

Although I knew Marj for all of a half hour, it seemed apparent that she was battling to hold back considerable emotion and was losing the battle. I suggested that her upset was about more than just this recent relationship.

Marj acknowledged that she was very sad. She could not understand why she had devoted twenty-five years to a marriage in which she did not belong. She was saddened that she would have no children. It was painful for her to hold someone else's baby. She felt she had wasted her life and was now too old.

It was understandable why Marj was trying to block out these emotions. If she felt them, would she fall apart? However, if she refused to feel them, would her blood pressure climb further and would she fall apart anyway? I explained that although she was afraid of these emotions, I didn't think feeling them meant she was falling apart.

I could see two directions to go. One would be to block out the distress with the help of tranquilizers or antidepressants and to treat the hypertension with pills. The other would be to feel the distress, with support, and begin the healing process. After all, she was forty-nine, not eighty-nine.

Marj very quickly chose the course of going with her emotions, however painful. I referred her to a psychotherapist, where she began to confront how she had always tried to please the men in her life, looking after their concerns but not her own. She began to uncover the roots of this attitude in her childhood.

Her blood pressure fell to normal and I discontinued her medication two months later. She will undoubtedly be confronted by more distress in the future and the choice of whether to face it. ◄

Marj's hypertension can be explained by her battle against feeling her emotions. When finally face-to-face with them, she was seeing herself as falling apart when she was actually opening the door to healing from her deep wounds. Avoiding the distress might work in the moment, but it cannot lead to healing.

Marj found that she was capable of facing the emotions she was avoiding without falling apart. However, there are more and deeper emotions yet to face. I believe she can avoid a lifetime of tranquilizers, antidepressants, and antihypertensive drugs by trusting herself to face her emotions instead of trying to pretend they aren't there. However, it won't be easy.

IRONICALLY, the best way to reduce the emotional discomfort we struggle to avoid, which can affect blood pressure, is to feel it. However, instead we focus on avoiding the discomfort and feeling better, and we are encouraged to do so by friends and family. Avoiding emotions is a temporary fix for a problem that will recur and recur until its roots are acknowledged.

It takes courage to acknowledge that which we have not wished to feel. I have encountered many patients who tell me they feel fine and that everything is okay in their life, when their life is obviously not okay. They are unwilling to acknowledge, or come to grips with, major problems in their life.

We often prefer to live a lie, feeling safer if we insist that everything is okay, or believing that nothing can change anyway. If we take a harder look, we might have to acknowledge that something is wrong. We can create changes in our lives if we have the courage to recognize when there is a problem.

As summarized by Roger Dafter, our negative emotions have positive value for us. They serve us, when we pay attention to them. Our distress is the signal that motivates us to make changes, if we are willing to face it.

Heeding Our Emotions

▶ Rhonda, forty-eight, was worried about her blood pressure. In my office, it was slightly elevated, but it averaged a normal 122/72 on a twenty-four-hour monitor.

To avoid hypertension, Rhonda was pursuing a healthy lifestyle, albeit to an extreme. She was very thin, did not smoke, jogged several miles every day, was a vegetarian, and consumed no salt.

Ironically it was because of her zeal to avoid blood pressure elevation, which she didn't have, that she felt unwell. She was tired all the time. I suspected she was fatigued because she ran too much and because her diet did not replenish the salt she lost in sweating. Her vegetarian diet contributed to iron deficiency. Being quite thin, she was also a candidate to develop osteoporosis. I recommended calcium and iron supplements, and also suggested that she run less and eat more salt.

She returned a year later. She was eating more salt and taking the supplements. Although less fatigued, she was now complaining of palpitations. She indeed had extra beats, a condition that is not uncommon and usually is not harmful or dangerous. A heart rhythm monitor identified the premature beats as benign.

Rhonda's concern about her extra beats had replaced her concern about her blood pressure. I began to wonder if there was a more serious concern in her life that she was ignoring or avoiding. Yet she stated that she was happily married, had a son whom she adored, had no financial concerns, and was actually quite pampered. She said she did not have any emotional concerns.

She returned a year later with a new and more serious problem. For four months she had had almost daily attacks of weakness and dizziness. Her blood pressure, normal at other times, would increase to 170/100 during the attacks. The attacks came on suddenly and were unrelated to stress. They would last two hours and leave her exhausted. Her life had come to a halt as she was either having attacks, recovering from them, or waiting in fear of the next one.

Tests excluded a pheochromocytoma, a tumor of the adrenal gland that can cause episodic hypertension, as described in Chapter 7. With her life coming to a halt, I decided to search with Rhonda for emotions that she might not be feeling, which I suspected had been the problem all along, in her obsession about her health.

She could identify no current stress other than her health. She had experienced no overt trauma. Her childhood had been an average one, with parents who were neither abusive nor particularly affectionate.

I asked again about her current life. She insisted she had a life most women would love to have. Pampered, affluent. I asked her if she was happy. She said yes. . . . Well, pretty happy. . . . Well, not that happy. . . . . Well, actually quite miserable.

She began to cry and told me she was ashamed of herself. She had avoided feeling that shame for decades, preferring to believe she was happy. She was ashamed because she had no purpose in life. Everyone she knew had a goal in their activity. She had none.

She had mentioned these feelings to no one, and had managed to avoid and even forget them. Yet I could sense her pain, the bind she was in.

Sitting in my office, she felt very sad, yet somewhat better. The secret was out. For the first time, I felt a sense of connectedness with her, instead of the barrier of her anxiety that I had always felt between us.

Her physical health had never been the problem. Acknowledging her emotions, her condition now made sense to her and to me. Rhonda felt lost, but for years she had lacked the motivation to do anything about it because she had not acknowledged her discontent.

The attacks ceased that same day and never recurred. I referred her to a psychotherapist.

She returned a year later for a checkup. Although she had not liked the psychotherapist and had quickly stopped seeing her, the anxiousness she always felt in the past was gone and she had stopped worrying about her blood pressure. However, she felt very depressed at times.

Her husband wanted her to be the bubbly wife she had always been, just as her parents had always wanted her to be the bubbly child and did not want to hear about her troubles. She told me she had seen a psychiatrist who told her that her depression was the result of a chemical imbalance. He prescribed an antidepressant. She felt better and was able again to avoid her emotions and be the smiling wife her husband wanted her to be. However, she chose to stop the medication and her sadness returned.

Rhonda remained off medication and her commitment to a healing process grew. Even without psychotherapy, she began to realize the truths her emotions were conveying to her, and the value of paying attention to them. She gradually felt less depressed. She did not feel up every day but realized that was okay. She took a part-time job and is continuing to change her life. ◄

We are responsible for the choices we make. Like many others, Rhonda had chosen to hide from her distress at how she was living her life. She had avoided making changes. The cost of hiding became greater and greater until finally it brought her life to a halt. Her physical symptoms, all along, were a clear signal that a change was needed. It was up to her to heed that signal.

Rhonda's family wanted her to "be happy," unwilling to accept that she was entitled to be unhappy at times. Only when she realized that feeling upset was appropriate and needed could she tolerate the distress and be guided by it.

▸ Ken, forty-six, had every reason not to have hypertension. He was thin and he exercised every day. His diet was low in salt and fat. No one in his family had hypertension. He enjoyed his white-collar job and had financial security. If anything, his work stress was less than ever.

Nevertheless, for the past six months most of his blood pressure readings, whether at the doctor's office or at his health club, were in the 150s/80s. Ken had read up on hypertension and had analyzed everything about his health, but he was not able to come up with an answer for why he had it.

My medical evaluation did not suggest anything other than essential hypertension, even though, as discussed in Chapter 10, Ken was exactly the type of person who shouldn't have it. His hypertension begged for an explanation. The stress in his life did not explain it. Without considering emotions he might have been avoiding, his hypertension would remain a mystery.

Ken was single and was not in a relationship at the time he saw me, but he wanted to marry someday. I asked him what had kept him from marriage until now. Partly, he said, it was because he had not met the right woman. Partly it was because he had been traveling so much up until the current year. Mostly, having grown up in a home with five children and not enough money, he wanted financial security before he married. However, he acknowledged he had achieved that financial security years ago. Quite simply, whatever the excuses, he was alone because he had chosen to be alone, and now, at some level, he was realizing that this choice might not have been the right one.

I asked Ken about his parents. Was he close to them? He answered yes, but I noted the pause before he answered. Ken's father, a blue-collar worker who could not keep up with the cost of raising five children, was a bitter and withdrawn man who became an alcoholic. He was not abusive or angry, just depressed and withdrawn. Seeing his father this way was what had motivated Ken to seek financial security.

I suggested to Ken that his blood pressure was a gauge of emotions inside him—emotions he might not be fully in touch with. Although he had sought and achieved his professional and financial goals, he had neglected the personal side of his needs, including the possibility of marriage and family, having chosen emotional isolation instead. His blood pressure was telling me that this was a bigger concern for him than he was allowing himself to realize. At forty-six, it was time to put his personal life in order.

I asked Ken his reaction to my thoughts. He acknowledged that in his gut that's how he felt. However, facing the absence of a personal life, rather than filling all his time with work as he had done, was scary. He had felt better ignoring the distress that was stirring. Ignoring it, he was also ignoring the impetus to create change in his life. The consequences of avoiding recognition of the crisis in his life were now beginning to appear.

Ken acknowledged the crisis in his life. He began to address his self-neglect through group process, as I will describe in the next chapter. Although his problem will not disappear overnight, his blood pressure has fallen and is consistently around 130/70, both at the gym and in my office. He has avoided the need for medication, instead choosing to examine how he is living his life. ◄

Our nature is to evolve as we go through life. If we do not, if we seek to do exactly the same things decade after decade, we are defying our nature. This can eventually lead to a life crisis when we realize that what once worked for us no longer works.

When that life crisis occurs, we can heed it, feel the distress, and create change in our life and relationships. Some will succumb to the distress and get depressed rather than realize the opportunity for change and the positive value of that distress. Still others will avoid the life crisis by keeping busy and paying no attention to the stirring within.

We can avoid the distress this way, and if our blood pressure rises, we can see a doctor and receive medication that will work. Then we can continue to ignore the alarms going off in our mind and body. We avoid looking inside and acknowledging that deep down something is wrong.

Hypertension often provides the signal that we are refusing to look inside. We can choose to heed it or to view it as a physical condition with no other meaning.

Perhaps your hypertension has such a meaning or perhaps it is a physical condition with no meaning. How can you tell which is the case? You can tell by looking at your life. Are you hiding from a major problem? Is there a major problem that should be bothering you but isn't? Your hypertension might be a clue that something is wrong. Don't ignore that clue.

Yes, It Is Emotion Based, and, No, You're Not Crazy

Many people are very reluctant to consider the possibility that their hypertension or other physical condition is linked to emotions. To many, acknowledging an emotional link implies emotional weakness. The following story offers a powerful lesson of the fallacy and harm of such a view.

> ▸ Irene, fifty, had suffered from depression in the past, but on a high dose of antidepressant medication the depression had improved. In the past eight years, her condition was dominated instead by physical illness. She suffered episodic hypertension, a syndrome described in more detail in Chapter 7. Her systolic blood pressure often exceeded 200 at these times. She suffered episodes every two weeks, tied to her menstrual cycle, and they left her exhausted. She had reached the point of medical disability.
>
> I was asked to evaluate Irene's hypertensive episodes after she was admitted to the hospital because of the chest pain accompanying

an episode. Tests showed she was not having a heart attack. Her history and previous tests that had excluded a pheo strongly suggested that her hypertension had a basis in hidden emotions.

Irene had seen many doctors over the years. Some had suggested an emotional basis for her condition, but Irene was infuriated at this suggestion. Being forewarned, I was not optimistic about her willingness to consider a mind–body connection.

Finding trauma in her history was not hard. She had been physically abused by her mother and sexually abused by her father. She had also been physically abused by her former husband.

I described to her how I had seen many patients with attacks exactly like hers and that many had improved. She listened attentively, looking for hope. I described how most of the patients I saw with this disorder had a history of trauma and how blocking their most painful emotions had enabled them to survive through very difficult times.

Irene could easily agree that she had suffered severe trauma. She understood that she had hidden much of the emotions related to it. I told her that I viewed her as a victim of torture and trauma rather than of emotional illness—of a personal nightmare that was extraordinarily harsh.

Irene always knew she was a survivor of torture, but it had never occurred to her that her physical condition could be a consequence of it. Whereas she had been vehemently opposed to blaming her physical condition on an emotional problem, she could readily see it as the post-traumatic disorder that it was.

When I told her I saw her as a survivor of torture, something hit home. She felt I understood her life story and its effect on her. Rather than refusing to consider this mind–body origin, she immediately understood and embraced it. For the first time, her physical illness made sense to her.

When I left, she told me she was happy. This abused woman, whose life had come to a halt, said she felt understood.

Irene's attacks virtually ceased. She began to see a psychotherapist at New York Hospital who specializes in treating the effects of trauma. She is aware of sadness emanating from her past, but, in her words, for the first time she also feels compassion for herself. She is healing and she knows it. ◂

When I discuss the mind–body connection of hypertension with my patients, one of the hardest things to convey is that "yes, there is a basis in hidden emotions, and, no, you're not crazy." Many patients describe to me how, when evaluated by a psychotherapist, they feel they are being cubbyholed into a diagnostic category. They don't like it. They feel as if they are being judged, that the psychotherapist is deciding what is wrong with them.

There are many fine psychotherapists who don't contribute to patients feeling this way. There are many who do, and I believe it is a huge barrier in healing.

When I listen to patients like Irene, I wonder how I would have survived had I lived through what she did. I suspect many of the patients I see have survived better than I might have. They survived; they are not emotionally weak.

I cannot "heal" them, but I can support them in their self-healing. I can witness their strength.

THE SHIFT OF AWARENESS, the mere recognition that we are affected by emotions we have hidden, can often by itself quickly promote healing of hypertension. Acknowledging our unwanted emotions rather than continuing the fight to keep them out of our awareness can enable us to replace illness with health.

The two biggest barriers to this awareness are our failure to realize our lack of awareness and the isolated manner in which many of us deal with our most painful emotions. Until we realize and address our isolation from our emotions and from each other, we will have little alternative to drugs in our treatment of hypertension and so many other conditions whose origin we cannot otherwise explain.

I have seen a sustained fall in blood pressure, or resolution of physical symptoms, occur in many patients even before the emotional work is begun. It is unclear to me what it is that produces this rapid effect. For some, like Ken, it may be the sharing with someone, for the first time, of concerns they have been struggling, successfully or unsuccessfully, to ignore. For others, like Irene, it may be the feeling of being understood. For others, like Roberta, it may be the mere telling for the first time of a long-forgotten story that could not be laid to rest before it was told.

Finally, for some, it may be the realization, for the first time, that what we have successfully endured can affect us and that we can safely face that which we once had to hide. A shift in awareness of our concealed emotions can heal hypertension and can also begin the process of emotional and spiritual healing. Some of the resources that can help in this process are described in the next chapter.

CHAPTER 12

Getting the Help You Need

T HE FIRST STEP IN THE HEALING PROCESS, the recognition that we are affected by emotions concealed within us, can sometimes quickly lead to improvement in blood pressure and other physical health problems. It also opens the door to begin a second process—the longer and more difficult process of emotional healing.

Opening Up to Hidden Painful Emotions

Addressing the true mind–body link is not simple. The healing process is often difficult and painful, which is why many people do not choose this path or even allow themselves to recognize their need for it. The case histories in this book reflect this reality. Nevertheless, I believe many people can benefit from having the choice of awareness.

With awareness, we open the door to feeling, and finally healing from, the terror, despair, or grief we have been hiding, perhaps for decades. In dealing with past emotional trauma we heal not by gentle reminiscence but by feeling the distress in the present while recognizing its origin in the past. However, often past and present become blurred during this process.

Our perspective and capacities as an adult, and the knowledge that we have survived, enable us to better tolerate these emotions. We are, in a way, playing a trick on time, experiencing the emotions of the past with the comfort of knowing that the future is okay.

Sharing these emotions with someone who honors rather than tries to abort the pain aids this process. Unfortunately, for many, this type of support is unavailable. Even worse, we tend to fear we are falling apart if we let in these emotions. The realization that feeling them is part of a healing process, rather than a sign of deterioration, is important in buttressing our willingness to face rather than avoid the emotions that are beginning to appear.

The emotional burden that some people are avoiding is a large one. The healing process can take weeks or months, or longer, and is never truly complete. Fortunately, not every emotion needs to be uncovered or needs to be felt right away.

During recovery, periods of severe distress can be interspersed with periods of calm, similar to the way grieving takes place. The distress may feel as if it will last forever, but it does not. Similar to grieving, we are mourning what has happened to us and we unknowingly design our unique schedule for feeling and discharging the emotions we have kept from awareness.

It is easy to lose sight of the light at the end of the tunnel. It is easy to forget that the distress is an unavoidable part of healing rather than a sign of breakdown. It is natural to seek to avoid rather than confront the distress. To heal, we need to know at a gut level that we can handle our difficult emotions, and then choose to face them.

There are many resources that can help in this healing process. I would like to briefly comment on some that have helped many people achieve awareness and acceptance of their deeply held emotions and that I therefore believe hold promise in the holistic treatment of hypertension and other medical disorders. They can help us relearn how to feel our emotions and to handle those that surface.

There are various forms of psychotherapy, group process, and meditation. The support available in spirituality, confiding, and connectedness is also extremely important in nurturing the healing process. Finally, medication, if needed, can play an important role. The variety of resources available attests to the widespread search for emotional healing and to the emotional scars so many of us bear. It also attests to the reality that no single resource is best suited for everybody.

There are many ways to find the right resource. Many excellent books have been written about recovery and personal growth and are available in personal growth and psychology sections in most bookstores. Recent best-selling books by John Bradshaw, Scott Peck, and Deepak Chopra are only a few. Information is also available on the Internet through search words such as *self-help, recovery groups, personal growth, self-awareness, mental health,* and *spiritual growth.* And, of course, friends who have themselves entered a healing process can provide valuable information.

There is no easy map to addressing the mind–body link of hypertension. The focus for decades on the readily apparent distress that we easily feel has raised false hopes of easy solutions and, for the most part, has not led to effective treatment. Approaches to treatment based on addressing hidden emotions have not been explored. I believe it is time to begin that task.

Emotional Awareness: Ways to Get Help

Psychotherapy, group process, and other techniques are valuable resources in the healing process. However, as I've discussed, they are most helpful once the first step, that of awareness, has opened the door.

Psychotherapy

Psychotherapy is not widely used in treating hypertension. A major barrier to its use is that people whose hypertension is driven by hidden emotions don't seek psychotherapy because they don't feel distressed. The cost and length of time required, and the lack of assurance of benefit, also discourage people from considering psychotherapy. Finally, the ease of controlling hypertension with a pill or two a day discourages it. Nevertheless, if the severity of your hypertension or the symptoms or pattern associated with it suggest an emotional basis, as I've discussed in Chapter 10, psychotherapy could be valuable.

People whose hypertension is linked to emotions they don't feel at all and which they insist are not affecting them do not tend to consider psychotherapy. They are also unlikely to benefit from it. As reported by Bonnie Strickland in 1963, and by others (see M. K. Thelen, 1969; and R. J. Pelligrine, 1971), people whose emotional distress is hidden from them are the most likely to prematurely terminate psychotherapy.

This is why I believe it is wrong to encourage people to enter psychotherapy for the sole purpose of treating hypertension unless they have achieved the important first step of realizing that their buried emotions are affecting them. Theresa, Martha, Marj, and others were able to utilize psychotherapy only after they began to realize the effects of emotions that had been hidden. Prior to that realization, psychotherapy would likely have been a waste of time.

Few studies have been performed to document the effect of psychotherapy in hypertension. Its role would be difficult to assess since, as described by Toksoz Karasu, there are over 450 types of psychotherapy in use, and since there are major differences from practitioner to practitioner. In addition, given the emphasis on pills and costs in contemporary medicine, it is unlikely that such studies would find support in the medical community.

I am often asked whether experiencing previously hidden emotions through hypnosis could be helpful in treating hypertension. It would seem unlikely. Experiencing hidden emotions in the altered state of hypnosis does not integrate them into conscious awareness, and I would therefore doubt that this alone would lower blood pressure. There is also cause for concern, as discussed by Bessel Van der Kolk in his book, *Traumatic Stress. The Effects of Overwhelming Experience on Mind, Body and Spirit* (1996), because evoking traumatic memories under hypnosis may also retraumatize patients. For these reasons I cannot recommend hypnotherapy, except perhaps as an adjunct to other forms of therapy.

Psychotherapy is both an art and a science. Its success depends on the unique skill, personality, and experience of the practitioner, and the fit between practitioner and patient, more than it does on the techniques used. It also depends on the patient's awareness and openness to searching within. Given the often formidable defenses against awareness in individuals whose hypertension is driven by their hidden emotions, the success of psychotherapy is far from assured.

TWO ADDITIONAL FACTORS are extremely important to the success or failure of psychotherapy. One is the distinction between knowing about versus feeling the emotions related to important events in our lives. The other is the attitude of the psychotherapist.

Knowing versus feeling. I have encountered many people who spent years in psychotherapy, and understood very clearly their history and its effects on them. Their understanding, however, did not lead to improvement in their physical or emotional symptoms. How can this be so?

The answer lies in the crucial distinction between knowing (intellectual) and feeling (emotional). When patients tell me that they barely shed a tear during years of psychotherapy it is a telltale sign that they have talked about their emotions without truly feeling them. They may understand the emotions that haunt them, but they remain victimized by them.

Discussing deeply buried emotions without feeling them achieves understanding but not healing. A psychotherapist's interpretation of your past, no matter how accurate, does not bring about healing. In those cases where I have seen hypertension resolve, it has been because patients truly felt, rather than just understood, the emotions they had blocked from their awareness.

The attitude of the psychotherapist. When an emotional link to hypertension is suggested, some people feel accused of having something wrong with them, of having an emotional weakness. I do not feel that this is the case. I find that hypertension is linked to emotions more in people who have survived very difficult times by blocking their emotions when they needed to than in the victims who did not and suffered greater emotional consequences.

A healing process is not about finding out what is wrong with us. It is about finding out what is innately right and about our ability to heal ourselves. A good psychotherapist will recognize and trust a person's innate self-healing capacity and assist that process. I agree with Andrew Weil, author of several books including *Spontaneous Healing*, that we harbor an innate tendency to self-healing. This is what a good psychotherapist will tap into.

Some psychotherapists unfortunately view their patients as flawed individuals who need their expert advice and skillful intervention in order to heal, and they relate to them accordingly. They trust their skill and techniques more than the patient's innate ability to heal. This can damage rather than foster a patient's self-trust, self-respect, and self-healing ability. A therapist with this view is likely to be the wrong psychotherapist for you.

I often encounter people who revere a psychotherapist and are very dependent on him or her. While a healthy therapeutic dependence might temporarily be necessary or even desirable, excessive or prolonged dependence is a red flag that your innate strength is not being tapped. Ultimately, good psychotherapy should promote self-trust rather than overreliance on others.

Group Process

When we handle our most painful emotions in isolation, we are more likely to need to avoid them rather than face them openly. Opening up to painful emotions is hard to do without solid human support. Studies and common sense tell us that people enjoy better health and feel better when receiving the emotional support of caring people. Many of us lack this healing connection and might be unaware of its absence.

Experience in an environment of emotional connectedness can help break the grip of this isolation. This kind of environment can be found in many group processes that have proliferated throughout the country. Their value has been demonstrated with the twelve-step programs that have succeeded in helping people overcome substance abuse and other problems, where traditional medical models have failed. In recent years, group processes have evolved to both promote healing and break down the barriers that isolate us from ourselves and from others. They provide powerful experiences that can encourage sustained life changes.

In group psychotherapy or group workshops, careful attention is given to the creation of an atmosphere of acceptance, safety, connectedness, and openness, conditions that are often absent from our day-to-day lives. This experience fosters the realization that our fundamental state is one of connectedness rather than the state of alienation and separateness that seems normal to many of us.

The experience of belonging and respect, and the willingness of participants to confront and confide their distressing emotions, encourages an openness and bonding that can be a powerful healing factor. Such workshops can foster in participants awareness of painful emotions buried as long ago as childhood.

A powerful feature of some group workshops is the period of time they provide away from the external concerns that otherwise dominate our attention. Rather than a mere hour stolen from a busy routine, many workshops provide two or more days away, with people who are equally committed to the process of self-awareness and change.

Many programs assist recovery from the lifelong effects of childhood abuse and trauma. These include groups for survivors of physical and sexual abuse, incest, adult children of alcoholic parents, and many others. Some groups nurture our lost connection to spirituality. Others provide support during periods of grief. Still others focus on personal growth, with attention to dealing with blocked emotions and building of self-esteem and connectedness. There are support groups for many medical, emotional, and addictive disorders. Recently, the benefit of such a support group was demonstrated in improved survival in women with metastatic breast cancer (see D. Spiegel, 1989).

Group workshops provide an environment in which people who are not accustomed to feeling and sharing deeply painful emotions can truly feel them rather than just talk about them. Others, however, might feel more comfortable in the one-on-one setting of psychotherapy. Group workshops can also be of value in combination with psychotherapy. Psychotherapy can enhance the effectiveness and safety of group process, while group process can accelerate the progress attained in psychotherapy.

The value of group processes in treating hypertension or other physical conditions that result from our isolation from our emotions has not been established, because their use for this purpose has not been widely considered or studied. However, since group process enables people to address hidden emotions and emotional isolation, they target precisely the emotional component of hypertension. I have come across two studies reporting that group psychotherapy led to a fall in blood pressure (see R. Peled-Ney, 1984; and K-D. Haehn, 1985). However, further documentation of this benefit is needed.

Evidence for the benefit of group process in mind–body disorders can also be found in the pioneering work done by Dr. John Sarno, and his associate, Dr. Arlene Feinblatt, in treating people with back pain. Data collected over years of workshops show that Feinblatt's eight-session group workshops, in which she confronts participants' tendency to block awareness of emotions, resulted in improvement in back pain in 65 percent of 137 people. A similar approach for treatment of hypertension and other mind–body disorders warrants study.

The process of undoing decades-old patterns obviously is not completed overnight, and the effects of a single workshop will fade without continued nurturing. For this reason, at the Hypertension Center I have begun to explore the effects of a series of weekend workshops in sustaining the impetus for awareness and change. It has been my privilege to work with Charles Bloom, a psychotherapist and enormously talented and experienced group facilitator, who runs the workshops. The workshops have helped participants focus on the importance of paying attention to their emotions. Further assessment of the impact of this type of intervention on hypertension is needed.

In a recent study, funded by the Fan Fox Foundation, I investigated the effect of a weekly two-hour workshop on blood pressure in people above the age of sixty-five. In this pilot study, participants ended up with a systolic blood pressure that was on average 5 millimeters lower than that of a control group that did not attend the workshops. Interestingly, the blood pressure of participants who were living alone fell, on average, 5 to 8 millimeters, while that of married participants were unchanged. This result suggests, as I will discuss, the importance to our health of close personal contact with others.

IT MAY SEEM ODD that sometimes we have to meet with strangers in order to learn to be more emotionally intimate. However, if we are alone, or if we don't confide in those around us and are unaware of connectedness, we may need to move outside our usual environment to learn a different way. We can then bring this powerful experience back into our relationships with family and friends.

Behavioral/Cognitive Techniques
Various relaxation techniques, anger and stress management techniques, biofeedback, and meditation can help in managing emotional distress. Meditation in particular is widely practiced as a means of both relaxation and self-awareness.

However, as I discussed in Chapter 3, relaxation techniques, anger and stress management techniques, and biofeedback have been found to have little persisting effects on blood pressure, and therefore cannot be recommended as an important treatment for hypertension. Charles Alexander reported in 1996 that meditation led to a sustained 10 millimeter lowering of blood pressure, although further studies are needed to confirm this result.

A recently developed and intriguing technique is rapid eye movement desensitization (EMDR) as described by Francine Shapiro in her book, *EMDR: The Breakthrough Therapy for Overcoming Anxiety, Stress, and Trauma*. She discovered quite by accident that rapid eye movements can bring hidden emotions into awareness, and diminish their impact. It has already become a treatment of choice for post-traumatic stress disorder. The possible role in treating hypertension of this and other techniques believed to facilitate access to hidden emotions is unknown.

Medications

Hidden emotions are often extremely painful ones and getting in touch with them in the healing process can produce severe distress. We did not hide those emotions without reason.

Fortunately, many excellent drugs are available, if needed, to assist in handling that distress. A variety of antidepressant and antianxiety agents can reduce the severity of emotional discomfort during very painful parts of the healing process. They can also relieve physical manifestations of hidden emotions, such as those associated with episodic hypertension, as discussed in Chapter 7. Many of these symptoms cannot be relieved by antihypertensive drugs.

In instances in which past trauma is severe and the hidden emotions that are causing difficult problems are truly too overwhelming to be confronted, these medications might be the only means to provide relief. Unfortunately, because the symptoms are physical, the use of these medications often is not even considered.

As with any drug, side effects are possible, but fortunately they are rarely dangerous. Another concern is that medications can be misused as a quick fix. In eliminating emotional or physical distress, they can reduce the impetus for self-exploration. Rhonda, whose story was discussed in the previous chapter, faced exactly this temptation.

Just as the optimal treatment of hypertension involves the use of both drug and nondrug therapies, navigating through the healing process also involves choices. I prefer to avoid medications where possible, but believe the failure to use them when needed and appropriate is also wrong. Pharmacologic advances are an important component of holistic care when they are used to support, rather than substitute for, a healing pathway.

Confiding, Connectedness, and Spirituality

Confiding, connectedness, and spirituality are vitally important resources in enabling us to face and tolerate our emotions, yet they are often sorely missing. Many people are not even aware of their absence and of the strength we can derive from them.

In an age of powerful and increasingly expensive drugs, connectedness and confiding are the cheapest, most abundant, and most underused weapons we have in mitigating the physical and emotional consequences of the emotions we avoid. Instead, most of us withdraw into ourselves when we most need to reach out.

Many societal conditions contribute to the limited role of confiding and connectedness. Many of us were raised in families where these were not experienced. Unfamiliar with these resources, we are also unaware of their absence.

Our geographic mobility cuts down on lifelong friendships and family ties. The extended family has waned as a uniting force. Unsatisfying marriage and divorce are more the rule than the exception. Perhaps most important, we cannot confide when we, and those around us, seek reflexively to halt emotional pain rather than come together to acknowledge it.

The Power of Confiding

I am surprised how often my patients acknowledge to me that although they are surrounded by friends and family, they always handle their deepest distress alone. They might discuss minor day-to-day problems, but they handle their most overwhelming issues by themselves by not letting the distress "get to them."

This state of emotional isolation is epidemic and we don't even realize it. Unfamiliar with any other way of being, we accept this state as normal, not realizing there is another way. Instead, we seek treatment for the physical and emotional consequences of that isolation and complain of the unwieldy health care costs that result.

Many of us learned this way of living as far back as childhood, when obtaining relief by talking with others was not available. Instead, as discussed in Chapter 6, we learned to block out the emotions. Feeling okay, we don't see the need to confide our emotions in anyone.

Over the years many patients have discussed extremely painful topics with me. At first, both the patient and I were afraid the discussions would trigger sky-high blood pressure readings. After all, James Lynch, in research he describes in his book *The Language of the Heart*, documented that when people speak about emotionally "hot" topics their blood pressure can soar. However, I found that after patients felt and shared with me emotions they had shared with no one, their blood pressure readings did not increase; they often fell. Seeing this demonstrated to me the power of confiding.

Why did the blood pressure soar in Lynch's studies, yet often fall in my office? I suspect that the difference lies in the setting—a physiologic experiment versus intimate conversation. I once hooked up a monitor to measure patients' blood pressure during such conversations. The factual content of the conversation was unchanged, but the emotional content and the mutual sense of connectedness were gone. With the monitor, our focus drifted to the effect of our conversation rather than to each other; there was no sense of intimacy. This is why I believe the effect of confiding cannot easily be documented in a laboratory. The personal connection is key.

The healing effect of confiding depends on the true sharing of emotions in an emotionally connected way. Ironically, the expression of emotional distress is sometimes a barrier rather than a bridge to connectedness and to the sharing of deeper feelings. I believe this occurs when people feel their distress in an emotionally isolated way, truly unfamiliar with sharing emotions. Regardless of the reason, the inability to confide is a barrier to easing distress. Recognizing this is an important step in the path to healing.

There are many reasons why many of us do not confide our most distressing emotions in anyone, even if married or surrounded by family and friends. We may feel that those around us have their own problems and we do not wish to upset them. Or perhaps others depend on us and we cannot show our "weakness," our own distress.

Perhaps we have no one with whom we feel comfortable enough to share our deepest distress. Perhaps we have always been unwilling, or too ashamed, to reach out to others. Perhaps we learned long ago that emotional distress is not something we share with others. Perhaps no one cares enough to listen. Perhaps they do, but we have trouble believing that they do.

Perhaps we never learned that confiding our distress can be comforting and can provide us with strength. Perhaps we simply don't know how.

Confiding is an often misunderstood term. It consists of simply communicating our feelings in an emotionally connected way and feeling a sense of relief after having done so. It differs from seeking advice or practical help. We much more easily reach out when we need help to carry a heavy carton, or need advice to solve a problem, but we less often do so when we have the much greater need to confide deep emotional pain.

The listener plays an important role in confiding. Offering advice or thinking about solutions connects the listener to his thoughts, not to the other person. *Simply listening, acknowledging a person's distress, and respecting his emotions is all that is needed.*

Confiding is not possible if the listener is trying to abort our distress. Too often at a time of emotional distress it is a knee-jerk reaction for a friend to try to make us feel better. Sometimes this is appropriate, but often it is not. If we are grieving after a death, for example, a friend who listens in a connected way and trusts and aids the grief process is more valuable than one who seeks only to divert us from that process.

Friends who fear and resist experiencing their own difficult emotions cannot support us in feeling and discharging ours. They will do their best to help us avoid rather than allow these emotions. The words "It's all right. Don't cry" are a barrier to confiding. True confiding means the acceptance that crying might be necessary.

You can bring the healing effects of confiding into your life simply by talking to someone you trust deeply, someone who is willing to listen without rushing to abort your distress. Group processes, as discussed, can also provide and teach confiding, and can bring its power into your life.

Connectedness

Connectedness is a mutual sense of attachment, even love. It is a sense of familiarity that transcends the isolation we often, and perhaps usually, feel. It is a state usually measured in minutes, not hours or days, yet carries with it enormous healing potential. Its healing power is unrecognized by many because we tend to be unaware of its absence in our life.

Its absence can easily go unnoticed. We certainly share good times with others and help each other solve problems. We often share common objectives and mistake that for connectedness. However, we often do not have or nurture the experience of connectedness, or seek the powerful support it provides.

I meet many people who have long known the value of connectedness with others in their life. They usually describe having had a childhood, whether happy or unhappy, in which they experienced a strong connectedness with family, or even a single member of the family, or someone outside the family.

I meet many others who have not known the value of connectedness. They might tell me they are not that kind of person or that they don't need it. They might not see its absence as a problem. They might not even be aware of its absence, since they never experienced it and therefore don't seek it.

It is important to bear in mind that the capacity for connectedness is innate to us, even if it seems foreign. In seeking it, we are seeking to take back that which is our birthright, that which resides within us even if we don't realize it. However, only when we first recognize its absence and recognize our right to it can we do something about it.

We cannot measure connectedness scientifically. Yet its value, social and psychological, if not medical, is obvious. The impact of its absence is suggested in a study reported by Lisa Berkman in the *Annals of Internal Medicine* in 1992, which showed that people who lack a network of emotional support were three times as likely as others to die in the first six months after a heart attack. William Ruberman similarly reported in the *New England Journal of Medicine* in 1984 that social isolation was associated with a doubling of mortality over a three-year period. Emotional isolation was the single most important factor in predicting mortality, outranking cholesterol level, smoking, and hypertension, among others.

A study by Linda Russek, published in 1997, reported that growing up feeling unloved was associated with physical illness in adulthood. She found that conditions such as coronary artery disease, hypertension, peptic ulcer disease, and alcoholism occur with increased frequency in adults who report having grown up in a home in which they did not feel loved. Feeling alone, they learned to hide from their emotions and to suffer the illnesses that result.

There are many barriers to connectedness. The biggest barrier is that we are unaware of its absence and therefore do not seek it. Another major barrier is that we are unaccustomed to focusing on the bonds that draw us closer to others. We might fear rejection. We might act in ways that prevent others from feeling connected to us.

The absence of the experience of connectedness is a condition we can do something about. Paying attention to the quality of our bonds with those around us and verbalizing our feelings to them can help advance this process. Group processes, as discussed previously, offer a powerful opportunity to learn to do this and to escape the isolation, both from others and from ourselves, that too many of us have come to accept as normal.

Faith and Spirituality

Psychotherapy has assisted many people in their healing process. However, it fails to help many others. In this setting, renewed attention is beginning to be directed at our spiritual wounds and spiritual needs. I believe a discussion of mind–body healing is incomplete without paying attention to their impact on our health.

IN SPIRITUAL PURSUIT we are seeking meaning in our lives beyond our external experience in the material world. We are seeking a unity with others, with the world around us, and with God, rather than the apartness that dominates our existence. Faith is the outcome of our search, and our faith helps us handle the stress of living and dying. Our faith provides meaning that helps us cushion the impact of the painful events we endure.

Polls report that 96 percent of Americans say they believe in God. I would suspect that many "sort of" believe in God. When I speak with patients, many describe the social and moral values of religious affiliation, but fewer mention the spiritual value and comfort of their faith.

Amid centuries of technological and social evolution, our spiritual awareness may actually have weakened. If anything, with our reliance on science to solve our problems, with the fast pace of life that occupies so much of our time with external concerns, and with the loss of a sense of community in crowded cities, we might have taken a step backward spiritually. As a result, the resilience that spirituality provides in times of stress is less available.

IN ADDRESSING THE MIND–BODY CONNECTION of physical illness, considerable attention has been paid to psychological interventions. The role of religion and spirituality has received much less attention. Many in the research and medical communities have considered it irrelevant to physical health. The founders of psychoanalytic therapy were strongly opposed to consideration of spiritual and religious values and their role in emotional healing. Psychotherapeutic methods developed outside of religious and spiritual circles.

At the same time, some religious communities shunned the value of psychotherapy, seeing it as a threat to the maintenance of religious traditions. Consideration of psychology and psychotherapy remains anathema in some religious communities, no matter how serious the emotional wounds in some of its members. In this fashion, many who promote a return to religion often remain blind to the need for emotional healing, while many proponents of psychotherapy similarly minimize the need for spiritual healing.

Fortunately, we are in an era when both psychology and religion are evolving. In many circles, the strong focus on unacceptable religious dogma is no longer central. The passion for spirituality is growing rapidly. Similarly, the disregard, and even disdain, for religion held by many in the psychotherapeutic community is being challenged and overturned.

I believe we are finally beginning to realize that spiritual and emotional healing are inseparable. Their combined impact may be exactly what we need if we are to escape the physical and emotional effects of our spiritual and emotional wounds.

I believe optimal healing involves attention to both our spiritual and emotional wounds. Perhaps this is why seeking emotional healing through psychotherapy, while ignoring our missing spiritual connection, often falls short. Similarly, seeking spiritual healing while ignoring the emotional barriers to spirituality also fails to achieve healing and inner unity. Emotional healing is enhanced in the setting of a spiritual connection, while spiritual healing depends on recognizing the emotional wounds barring it.

Whether we are seeking to address spiritual wounds or emotional wounds, we face exactly the same problem: our lack of awareness that there is a problem. Just as we don't realize that something is missing in our lives when we are out of touch emotionally, we don't realize that something is missing when we are out of touch spiritually. We see a state lacking in spirituality as normal. We don't yearn for what we haven't tasted.

That is why the path to both emotional and spiritual healing often begins with, and requires, a shift in our awareness. It is this shift that opens the door to regaining the spirituality that many of us have never felt.

However, even with the door open, true spiritual healing does not come easily. It cannot be achieved solely through intellectual effort, no matter how intense. Many resources can help us in this struggle. Music, books on spirituality, affiliation with and support from a spiritually minded group or community, nurturing our relationships with others, setting aside time for contemplation, and performance of religious ritual can all be helpful in nurturing the spirituality that lies within us.

As this millennium draws to a close, I believe we are witnessing an evolution in both religion and psychology, one marked by recognition of their common goals rather than the disdainful view each has held of the other. With this unity, we can hope for greater strides in achieving mental and physical health. Our inability to cure so many medical conditions argues for such a union.

Choosing the Best Medication

IDENTIFYING AND ADDRESSING HIDDEN EMOTIONS offers a way to lower blood pressure and lessen or eliminate the need for medication. However, even when a source in hidden emotions can be identified, it is not always possible to avoid medication altogether.

Many people will not accept that they harbor and are affected by emotions they do not feel. Some cannot and some should not engage those emotions. However, identifying whether their hypertension is emotion-based can be helpful in selecting the best drug or drugs to treat it.

What You Can Do Before Resorting to Medication

If I were to evaluate your hypertension in my office, I would undertake several tasks to determine its cause and the best means of treating it. My first task would be to establish whether you truly have hypertension or just a transient elevation of your blood pressure. If you truly have hypertension, I would seek to determine whether it is essential hypertension, as it is in over 95 percent of people with hypertension, or whether you are one of the few in whom there is a specific cause that can be identified and cured.

I would also assess whether your hypertension has damaged organs such as the heart, kidneys, or brain. If it has, I would err on the side of being more aggressive in treating your hypertension.

Assuming that you have essential hypertension, my next task would be to try to determine *why* you have it. Are you overweight and sedentary? Is salt a factor? Does everyone in your family have high blood pressure, suggesting a genetic basis? Is the cause related to hidden emotions?

My next task would be to determine if nondrug measures can control it. If they cannot, I would decide whether to initiate drug therapy. If you have other risk factors for cardiovascular disease in addition to your hypertension, such as an elevated cholesterol level, a history of smoking, diabetes, or a strong family history of heart attacks or strokes, I would be more inclined to treat even the mildest of hypertension. If you have none of these risk factors I would try to wait longer and see what happens without medication.

Unless your blood pressure is severely elevated—that is, above 180/110—there is usually time to recheck it without rushing to begin medication. There is unfortunately a common misconception that untreated hypertension puts people at a high risk of suffering a stroke at any moment. It does not. The risk of mild hypertension is incurred over years to decades, not weeks or months. Therefore, there is usually time to observe whether your blood pressure will fall on its own. As discussed in Chapter 2, it will fall on its own in up to a third of people with mildly elevated readings (140–160/90–100).

The Joint National Committee on the Detection, Evaluation and Treatment of High Blood Pressure recommends a three- to six-month waiting period during which nondrug remedies can be tried before resorting to medication. This guideline should be followed unless your blood pressure is severely elevated or you have another condition that requires more rapid control of your blood pressure (such as angina, heart failure, or other conditions), or there is evidence that your hypertension has already caused damage.

If drug treatment is necessary, my next task would be to select the drug that would be best for you. My final task would be to make sure that the drug is working and that you are not suffering from side effects.

Nondrug Measures

Millions of people with hypertension can be treated without drugs, particularly if their hypertension is mild and if a small decrease in blood pressure is all that is needed to restore it to normal. Many nondrug measures have been proposed. Some have been proven effective, whereas others seem to provide uncertain or at best slight benefit. Numerous other treatments are constantly being suggested, although there is not enough evidence to strongly recommend their use.

**Nondrug Measures with Established Benefit
in Lowering Blood Pressure**
- ► Weight loss
- ► Salt restriction (in people with salt-sensitive hypertension)
- ► Exercise
- ► Reduction of excessive alcohol intake
- ► Potassium supplementation if diet is potassium deficient
- ► Low-fat diet high in fruits and vegetables

Weight loss. Obesity is strongly associated with the development of hypertension. However, the mechanism by which it causes hypertension is unclear despite considerable research.

I see many patients who exercise regularly and consume a diet far better than mine, yet they cannot lose weight. The basis of their obesity is likely to be mostly genetic. Addressing their emotional concerns could be expected to be of little value in losing weight.

In many other obese individuals, emotional distress, whether felt or hidden, contributes to hypertension either directly through its effects on the brain and sympathoadrenal system (see below) or indirectly through its effects on appetite and weight.

STUDIES SHOW CONSISTENTLY that weight loss can lower blood pressure (see D. E. Schotte, 1990). Unfortunately, it is the uncommon person who achieves and sustains weight loss. Appetite suppressants can promote weight loss, but some can be addictive and others have been removed from the market because of possible health risks. Clearly, better means of achieving sustained weight loss are needed.

Salt restriction. Salt restriction has been shown to lower blood pressure in many studies, as reviewed in 1991 by Jeffrey Cutler. Salt restriction can also increase the effectiveness of most antihypertensive drugs.

However, it is a common misconception that everyone with hypertension should restrict their salt intake. Studies indicate that salt restriction will lower blood pressure in approximately one in three people with hypertension. In others, extreme salt restriction can actually be harmful and should be avoided. The response to salt restriction varies by race, being more likely to lower blood pressure in African Americans than in whites.

There is no test that can predict perfectly whose blood pressure will respond to salt restriction. You can do your own experiment and restrict your salt intake for a week or two and see if your blood pressure falls. Measurement of the hormone renin in the blood can also be a helpful guide, as I will discuss below.

The degree to which salt restriction will lower your blood pressure depends on how strictly you limit your salt intake. Adequate salt restriction requires effort. It requires paying attention to your diet every day. Most people seem to know that they should avoid canned and many frozen foods, and they add little salt at the table and in cooking. However, you also need to pay attention to the high salt content in bread and in food served in restaurants. Many restaurants will prepare foods without salt for you, but only if you ask them to do so.

Exercise. As recently reviewed by Robert Fagard in 1995 and by George Kelley in 1994, studies consistently demonstrate that regular exercise can lower blood pressure. When patients ask me which type of exercise is best for them, I answer that the type of exercise they enjoy doing is the right one. You are unlikely to maintain an exercise regimen if you hate the exercise. Choose what you enjoy—whether swimming, walking, jogging, or cycling—and stick with it.

People with hypertension have always been advised not to engage in weight lifting because of the rise in blood pressure while lifting. However, there is no evidence of harm caused by this transient rise. If anything, weight training may actually lower your usual blood pressure (see R. L. Wiley, 1992). Nevertheless, I would recommend moderation because of the considerable, albeit brief, increase in blood pressure while lifting. I would also advise against weight lifting if your resting blood pressure is considerably elevated.

Reduction of excessive alcohol intake. Just how excessive alcohol intake raises blood pressure is unclear, but we know it does. Partly it is the effect of alcohol on the sympathetic nervous system (see below), and partly it is the effect of withdrawal when alcohol levels subside. I suspect also that the emotions that drive people to excessive drinking play a role.

Reducing excessive alcohol intake can lower your blood pressure (see I. B. Puddey, 1987). If you have a history of abusing alcohol, complete abstention is best. Otherwise, a drink or two a day will not raise your blood pressure and might provide slight protection against coronary disease.

Potassium supplementation. Many studies have shown that potassium supplementation can lower blood pressure in individuals whose diet is deficient in potassium intake. Its benefit in people with an adequate intake of potassium is less clear. However, instead of taking potassium supplements, adhering to a better diet, including more fruits and vegetables, is a much healthier way to assure adequate potassium intake.

Healthy diet. I cannot emphasize enough the importance of a healthful diet: one low in fats and high in fruits and vegetables. A recent report by Lawrence Appel in the *New England Journal of Medicine* confirmed the value of this diet, referred to as the DASH (Dietary Approaches to Stop Hypertension) diet, in lowering blood pressure. The essentials of this diet can be obtained through Internet sites (http://www.bloodpressure.com/newrsch/wrdash.htm or http://dash.bwh.harvard.edu./research.html), or from the National Heart, Lung and Blood Institute, either by mail (NHLBI Information Center, P.O. Box 30105, Bethesda, Maryland 20824-0105) or by telephone (301/251-1222). Also key is avoidance of excesses, whether fats, sweets, or total calories. This type of diet can benefit your hypertension in several ways. Your salt intake is lower. Your potassium intake is higher. Your caloric intake is lower, facilitating weight loss.

These guidelines are beneficial even if you don't have hypertension. You can lower your cholesterol level, help reduce the development of atherosclerosis, and help reduce cancer risk.

HEALTHFUL NONDRUG INTERVENTIONS are always worth trying. If you have mild hypertension, these interventions may be all that is needed to normalize your blood pressure and avoid medication. If you have more severe hypertension, these interventions usually will not bring your blood pressure down to normal but can help reduce the amount of medication you will require.

Nondrug Measures with Less Clearly Established Blood Pressure–Lowering Effects

- ▸ Calcium and magnesium supplements
- ▸ Relaxation techniques
- ▸ Biofeedback
- ▸ Garlic
- ▸ Fish oil
- ▸ Other unproven alternative therapies

Many other remedies have been proposed and popularized, but their effectiveness is less unanimously accepted. A review by Christopher Silagy, published in the *Journal of Hypertension* in 1994, suggests that garlic is slightly beneficial. Similarly, a review by Martha Morris in 1993 concluded that fish oil can slightly lower blood pressure. Calcium supplementation is also believed by many to be helpful, although a recent review of studies by P. Scott

Allander, published in the *Annals of Internal Medicine*, reported a fall in blood pressure averaging a negligible 1 millimeter.

Since hypertension resolves spontaneously in a third of people with mild elevations, any remedy tried will appear to lower blood pressure in some people. For this reason, many people swear by remedies that have not been proven, or even ones that have been disproven in controlled studies. Unfortunately, the number of suggested remedies greatly exceeds the capacity of funded research to prove or disprove. Thus, there will always be alternative remedies that are not on this list that might be effective but await better documentation.

Selecting the Right Drug

We now have many safe drugs that lower blood pressure. With them, hypertension can be controlled in most people, and the cardiovascular risk of hypertension can be greatly reduced.

However, drugs are not the ideal answer. Minor side effects are often a problem. The expense over the years is substantial. People have to remember to take them every day. Further, even if people take them, the drugs do not always work.

Even with the availability of effective medications, the blood pressure of most people with hypertension is still not under control. I was surprised when Vicki Burt found in the National Health and Nutrition Examination Survey that only 27 percent of people with hypertension had achieved a blood pressure level in the desired range below 140/90.

Many factors underlie these disappointing figures. Some people are not taking medication because they are unaware that they have hypertension. However, more often, they are not taking medication because of the expense or side effects. In addition, there is still a widespread but mistaken belief that if we feel well the hypertension is not harmful. It is difficult to adhere to medication for decades, especially when there are no physical symptoms to remind us that we need it. Most of us also do not like being reminded daily that we have a potentially dangerous illness.

Finally, in some individuals, hypertension truly cannot be controlled no matter what drug is taken.

The biggest limitation of drug therapy is that drugs are a treatment, not a cure. It is because they cannot cure that they must be taken for a lifetime.

THERE ARE SEVERAL WIDESPREAD BELIEFS about antihypertensive drugs that are unfounded. It is a mistaken belief that one medication lowers blood pressure more than any other. All seem to work in about 50 to 60 percent of patients. It is also unclear if treatment with any one drug saves more lives than treatment with any other. Some studies have suggested that calcium channel blockers may be less beneficial and that ACE inhibitors may be more beneficial, but definitive answers await the conclusion within the next few years of several large studies comparing the long-term outcomes of different drugs.

Another mistaken belief is that if all medications work in roughly the same percentage of people, a drug can be randomly selected. As reported by Stephen Attwood in 1994, an individual's response to a drug bears little relationship to how he will respond to other drugs. One drug might not affect your blood pressure, whereas another can be extremely effective.

It is a common error to think of hypertension as a single disorder with a single cause. Any number of causes can underlie it. Therefore, it is not surprising that a single drug does not work in everyone. Since each class of drugs lowers blood pressure by a specific mechanism, it is possible to optimize treatment by finding a drug that matches the mechanism of your hypertension. Logically, the drug that best addresses that mechanism is the one most likely to lower your blood pressure. The wrong drug is less likely to work and is perhaps more likely to cause side effects.

This logical approach is not widely promoted. The recent report of the Joint National Committee on the Detection, Evaluation and Treatment of High Blood Pressure does not promote the idea of selecting a drug according to the mechanism of the hypertension. Even in the current large multicenter studies that are comparing the effects of different drugs, these drugs are assigned to individuals on a random basis, as if the underlying mechanism of the hypertension were of no relevance to drug selection. There is little interest in who responded to which drug.

Physicians often select drugs based on their effects on conditions other than the hypertension being treated. Thus, a diuretic is prescribed for someone who has hypertension and fluid retention. Beta blockers are selected for people with hypertension and angina. Alpha blockers are selected for people who have hypertension and symptoms of an enlarged prostate gland. ACE inhibitors are prescribed in people with hypertension and kidney disease, to help protect kidney function. In this way, treatment kills two birds with one stone, although the drug is chosen independently of the mechanism of the hypertension.

Other reasons for selection of a drug focus on avoiding side effects. For example, we avoid using beta blockers in people with asthma, and diuretics in people with gout. However, in people without these conditions, and even in people with them, few physicians focus on the cause of the hypertension as a basis for drug selection.

Every physician knows that a given patient is likely to respond better to one drug than to another. The art of treating hypertension, therefore, lies in finding the right drug for each patient. The patient whose blood pressure seemingly cannot be controlled is usually simply on the wrong drug.

Brain Versus Kidney

Two organ systems have been shown to be intimately involved in the development of hypertension: the *brain* and the *kidney*. In some people hypertension is driven by the brain, in others by the kidney, and in still others by both. Most of the drugs that we use to treat hypertension are directed at one or the other of these two organs, as listed in the Appendix.

In this chapter I shall discuss how the brain and kidney are involved in the development of hypertension and how this information is pertinent to selecting the right drug or drugs. Many possible mechanisms are under study. Some have been proven to play a clear and important role in causing hypertension. The role of others is less clear. I shall focus on the most clearly established mechanisms, particularly those targeted by the antihypertensive medications in use today.

I believe we can tell whether your hypertension is predominantly driven by your brain and sympathetic nervous system by knowing whether hidden emotions are playing a role. In the best spirit of mind–body medicine, we can then optimize drug selection. I will begin by briefly explaining the major mechanisms by which the brain and kidneys affect your blood pressure.

Hypertension Driven by the Brain

The effects of emotions on blood pressure are mediated mainly by the *sympathoadrenal system*, which links the brain and brain stem to the cardiovascular system through two sets of nerves, as shown in Figure 13.1. One set, called the *sympathetic nervous system*, links the brain to the heart and arteries. The other, the *adrenal limb*, links the brain to the adrenal gland.

Stimulation of the nerves of the *sympathetic nervous system* raises blood pressure by constricting (narrowing) the arteries and veins, and by increasing the force of contraction of the heart. These effects are mediated through release at the nerve endings of the neurotransmitter *noradrenaline*, which binds to and stimulates receptors called *alpha receptors* located in the walls of the arteries and heart. Stimulation of these receptors triggers biochemical changes that cause smooth muscle contraction in the blood vessel walls, which narrows them and constricts the flow of blood through them. Usually we are unaware of constriction of our arteries, although at times we can sense it as coldness in our hands and feet.

The *adrenal glands*, one located above each kidney, secrete many important hormones into the bloodstream, including adrenaline, cortisol, and aldosterone. Stimulation of the nerves that

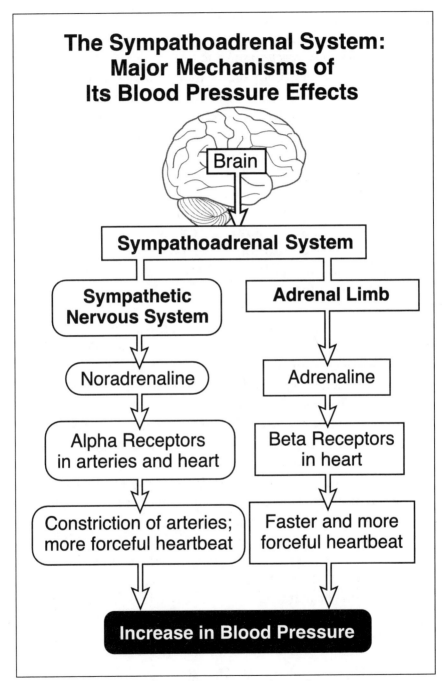

FIGURE 13.1. The two limbs of the sympathoadrenal system.

connect the brain to the adrenal glands increases their secretion of *adrenaline*. The adrenaline circulating in the bloodstream binds to and stimulates *beta receptors* in the heart. These activated receptors, in turn, increase both the heart rate and the force of contraction of the heart, and consequently the blood pressure. At times we can feel the effect of adrenaline in the rapid and forceful pounding of our heart. Adrenaline also stimulates beta receptors in the kidneys. These receptors increase the kidneys' secretion of renin, which also raises blood pressure, as I will discuss further in this chapter.

The brain also responds to stress in other ways. Its influence on secretion of the stress hormone cortisol by the adrenal glands and the effects of cortisol on blood pressure have been widely studied. To date the relationship between cortisol and essential hypertension remains unclear.

THE TWO LIMBS of the sympathoadrenal system normally help maintain our blood pressure in the normal range. The system is wired to act instantaneously to raise our blood pressure if it falls. For example, when we stand up and gravity pools more of our blood into the veins in our legs, the sympathetic nervous system constricts our blood vessels, limiting the amount of blood pooling and halting the fall in our blood pressure. The effects of this system wear off just as quickly.

The sympathoadrenal system also governs the fight-or-flight response that prepares us to cope with danger. It is responsible for the moment-to-moment fluctuation in our blood pressure associated with physical activity and with emotions.

Emotional distress can have varying effects on this system. Anxiety tends to stimulate secretion of adrenaline, which is why we can feel our heart racing when we are frightened. Anger tends to stimulate both limbs, causing our arteries to constrict and our heart rate to increase. Sadness also causes constriction of our arteries.

Control of the release of adrenaline was recently reviewed in *Stress, Catecholamines and Cardiovascular Disease* by David Goldstein. He points out that the release of adrenaline, although clearly associated with anxiety, does not require awareness of that anxiety. In other words, we can pump adrenaline even while insisting we feel calm. This matches exactly my experience with patients.

Anger or anxiety will raise anyone's blood pressure. This effect, however, is a temporary one, but one that can lead to the misdiagnosis of temporary blood pressure elevation as hypertension.

Many studies have shown that a sustained increase in the level of activation of the sympathoadrenal system is more common in people who have hypertension than in those who do not (see N. M. Kaplan, 1994; J. S. Floras, 1993; V. V. Panfilov, 1994; and M. Esler, 1987). Why it is more active is a mystery that has defied researchers for decades and continues to do so. One answer suspected by many is that individuals who have hypertension and who have increased activity of this system feel more angry or anxious than others. This tempting hypothesis, however, has not been borne out by research. Although the emotions we feel clearly do have temporary effects on this system and on blood pressure, most people with hypertension have not been found to be angrier or more anxious than anyone else.

I believe the emotions we have hidden from ourselves and that we battle to keep out of awareness can provide the missing explanation. Unlike the emotions we feel and discharge, these emotions persist within us and make more sense as an explanation for long-term sympathoadrenal activation. Unfortunately, this link has remained unexplored because these emotions cannot be measured and because most researchers are unaware of their potential role.

Clearly not everyone who has blocked very painful emotions will develop hypertension. There are several reasons for this. Aside from genetic predisposition, the effect of hidden emotions will depend on the magnitude of the incurred stress or trauma and on how powerfully the related emotions have been blocked. I suspect that deeply hidden emotions affect blood pressure less than emotions that are closer to the surface of awareness. Finally, weight, diet, and exercise further contribute to whether hypertension develops.

SEVERAL OF THE MOST WIDELY USED antihypertensive drugs work by blocking the effects of the sympathoadrenal system on blood pressure (see Appendix). The *beta blockers,* such as atenolol (Tenormin) and propanolol (Inderal), block the effect of adrenaline on the beta receptors in the heart. They do this by binding to those receptors, thus preventing adrenaline from binding to and activating them. Their most conspicuous manifestation is slowing of the heart rate, even in people without hypertension. The *alpha blockers,* such as prazosin (Minipress), terazosin (Hytrin), and doxazosin (Cardura), lower blood pressure by binding to the alpha receptors in the arterial walls, preventing noradrenaline from binding to them and causing constriction of blood vessels.

The *central alpha agonists,* such as clonidine (Catapres), act directly in the brain stem to reduce the level of activation of the sympathoadrenal system. They would seem ideal for treating hypertension driven by the brain, but unfortunately their effect is frequently accompanied by drowsiness and fatigue. Consequently, I avoid using them except when other drugs have failed. Two new drugs, moxonidine and rilmenidine, also work in the brain stem and might cause less drowsiness, but they are not available in the United States. They are safe and effective drugs and are available in Europe, but studies leading to Food and Drug Administration approval are needed.

Older and less commonly used drugs, such as reserpine (Serpasil) and guanethidine (Ismelin), also reduce activation of the sympathoadrenal system. Reserpine is actually a safe, inexpensive, and effective drug at the low doses currently employed. It lost favor because it caused depression at previously used higher doses, and because of studies linking its use to cancer—studies that were later disproven. Guanethidine often causes dizziness and/or diarrhea.

Several drug classes dilate constricted arteries via direct effects on the smooth muscle cells rather than through effects on the sympathoadrenal system. The calcium channel blockers reduce blood vessel constriction by closing the calcium channels through which calcium, which mediates smooth muscle contraction, enters these cells. The dihydropyridine type of calcium channel blockers, such as nifedipine (Procardia) and amlodipine (Norvasc), are powerful dilators. They are often given in combination with either an ACE inhibitor (see below) or a beta blocker. Other calcium channel blockers, such as diltiazem (Cardizem) and verapamil (Calan), dilate blood vessels and also slow the heart rate. Most calcium channel blockers can cause swelling in the legs. A recently approved calcium channel blocker, mibefridil (Posicor), is virtually devoid of this side effect, but has been at least temporarily removed from the market because of reports that it can cause a serious cardiac arrhythmia.

Recent reports have raised concern about the safety of the calcium channel blockers. A few reports suggest they may be less effective than other antihypertensive drugs in preventing heart attacks. Some studies report an increase in the risk of developing cancer. Others do not find this.

At this time, it is clear that short-acting dihydropyridine-type calcium channel blockers, such as nifedipine (Procardia), slightly increase the risk of heart attacks. The effect of long-acting calcium channel blockers on this risk, including Procardia XL, is unclear. Current multicenter trials will provide answers within the next few years.

Other vasodilators, such as hydralazine (Apresoline) and minoxidil (Loniten), are used less commonly because each, particularly minoxidil, speeds up the heart rate and can cause fluid retention. When either is used, a diuretic and beta blocker usually must also be given.

IN PATIENTS WHOSE HYPERTENSION appears linked to emotions, I generally prescribe beta blockers, alpha blockers, and dihydropyridine calcium channel blockers, either alone or in combination. The heart rate provides a useful aid to drug selection. An increased heart rate, above eighty or ninety beats per minute, suggests that adrenaline and beta receptors are prominently involved and that a beta blocker is likely to work either by itself or in combination with an alpha blocker. If the heart rate is slower, suggesting that vasoconstriction is a more important factor, I tend to prescribe a vasodilator such as an alpha blocker or calcium channel blocker, alone or in combination with a beta blocker. In patients with more severe hypertension, I usually initiate treatment with a combination of two drugs, that is, a beta blocker together with an alpha blocker or dihydropyridine calcium channel blocker, such as amlodipine (Norvasc). These combinations can lower blood pressure even when either drug by itself has little effect.

The combination of an alpha and beta blocker may be the best-suited combination to reduce the impact of emotions on blood pressure. Ironically, this combination receives far less attention than drug combinations involving newer drugs.

Hypertension Driven by the Kidneys: Understanding the Causes

Although the kidneys can affect blood pressure in many ways, the role of two factors has received the most attention in unraveling the mystery of hypertension: the *renin–angiotensin system* and *blood volume*. All of the available antihypertensive drugs that target the kidney attack one of these two mechanisms.

My former mentor at the Hypertension Center at the New York Hospital–Cornell Medical Center, Dr. John Laragh, did pioneering work concerning the reciprocal relationship between the renin–angiotensin system and blood volume in the normal regulation of blood pressure. His work produced evidence that renin measurement can help guide treatment of hypertension by matching the drug to the mechanism causing an individual's hypertension, as reviewed in an article by Dr. Laragh in 1989 in the journal *Hypertension*. I have used his approach for many years and have found it to be very helpful in selecting drugs, particularly for essential hypertension that is driven by the kidneys. I would like to briefly summarize that approach.

Our kidneys constantly assess whether our blood volume and blood pressure are at the right level based on the blood flow they receive. When the kidneys sense that either is slightly low—for example, if we have consumed little salt, have perspired a lot, or have taken a diuretic—they are programmed to decrease the salt and fluid we excrete into the urine and to increase their secretion of the hormone renin. The renin, in turn, as shown in Figure 13.2, stimulates the production of angiotensin I, which is converted by angiotensin-converting enzyme (ACE) to angiotensin II. Angiotensin II in turn binds to angiotensin receptors. Activation of these receptors causes arteries to constrict and also increases adrenal gland secretion of *aldosterone,* a hormone that reduces salt excretion by the kidneys. These effects help sustain blood pressure and avoid dehydration. Conversely, when blood pressure or blood volume is too high—for example, from consuming a lot of salt—our kidneys are programmed to secrete less renin and excrete more salt and fluid.

This reciprocal relationship between the blood volume and the renin–angiotensin system activation is depicted in Figure 13.3. If our blood volume is high, the blood renin level, which, unlike angiotensin, can be measured by a routinely available blood test, will be low, until the excess volume is eliminated. This is one reason why the excess salt in our diet normally does not elevate our blood pressure very much. Conversely, if our blood volume is a bit low, the renin level will be high.

Where we run into problems is either when we secrete more renin than we need to maintain a normal blood volume or blood pressure, or when we fail to excrete excessive salt and volume.

Hypertension Attributable to Excess Activation of the Renin–Angiotensin System

Overactivity of the renin–angiotensin system is the main cause of hypertension in perhaps a third of people with hypertension. Its cause has not yet been clarified, although genetic factors are believed important. Indeed, much research into the genetics of hypertension has focused on genes related to the renin–angiotensin system.

Activation of this system can also result from stimulation by circulating adrenaline of the beta receptors in the kidneys. Thus, when our bodies are pumping adrenaline, we are also stimulating renin secretion. Finally, in some people, excessive renin secretion

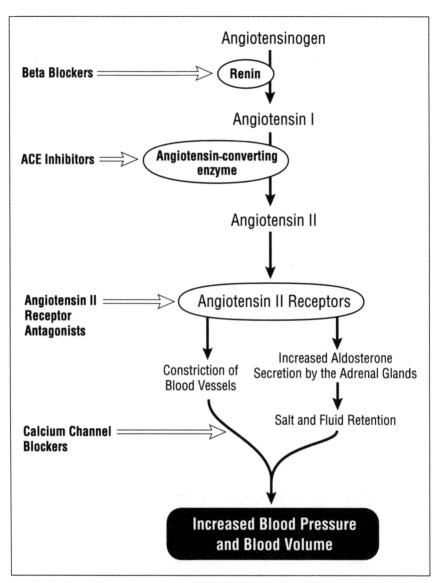

FIGURE 13.2. The renin–angiotensin system. The figure shows the steps that follow when renin secretion is stimulated by a reduction in blood volume or blood pressure. Also depicted are the steps at which various antihypertensive drugs interact with the renin–angiotensin system to oppose blood pressure elevation when excessive renin is causing hypertension.

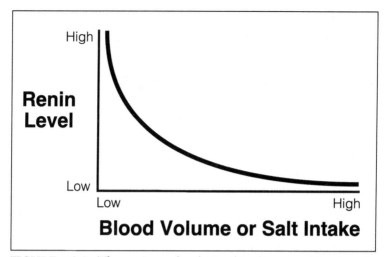

FIGURE 13.3. The reciprocal relationship between blood renin level and blood volume. The secretion of renin is stimulated when blood volume or salt intake is reduced. It is inhibited when they are increased.

can be a clue of hypertension caused by a narrowing of an artery to the kidney. Your physician can advise you as to whether a search for this condition is warranted.

Three widely used drug classes work well in hypertension caused by excessive activation of the renin–angiotensin system: the *ACE inhibitors,* which block the conversion of angiotensin I to angiotensin II; the *angiotensin II receptor antagonists,* which block the angiotensin II receptors in the arterial walls, kidneys, and adrenal glands; and the *beta blockers,* which suppress the secretion of renin by the kidneys by occupying the beta receptors otherwise bound by adrenaline.

The effect of ACE inhibitors and angiotensin receptor antagonists on blood pressure may also be related, to some extent, to blocking of the stimulating effect of angiotensin II on the sympathetic nervous system. Finally, an important advantage of the angiotensin receptor antagonists is their very low side effect profile.

A high renin level tells us that a beta blocker, ACE inhibitor, or angiotensin antagonist is likely to be effective, whereas other types of drugs, such as the diuretics, are not. When the renin–angiotensin system is driven by factors within the kidney, an ACE inhibitor or angiotensin antagonist will work best. When it is driven by adrenaline, a beta blocker might work better.

When hypertension of any cause is severe and longstanding, damage to, and narrowing of, the arteries supplying blood to the kidneys activates the renin–angiotensin system and further aggravates hypertension of any cause. At this stage of hypertension, treatment that blocks the renin–angiotensin system is often needed, even if it was not the initial cause of the hypertension.

Hypertension Attributable to Excess Volume
If the kidneys hold onto salt and volume too aggressively, blood volume and consequently blood pressure will increase. The increase in pressure is partly due to the increase in the volume of blood circulating within the arteries. It is also a result of an increase in the sodium ion concentration inside the smooth muscle cells that line the arteries. Through a mechanism called sodium-calcium exchange, this leads to increased calcium ion concentration inside these cells, which stimulates them to contract, thus constricting the blood vessels and raising blood pressure.

When blood is delivered to the kidneys at a higher pressure, the kidneys are better able to excrete the excess salt and volume. This is why people whose hypertension is caused by abnormal salt excretion do not become swollen with fluid. The kidneys do excrete the normal amount of salt and volume but only at the higher blood pressure.

The degree of tenaciousness with which our kidneys retain salt rather than excreting it is genetically conferred. It is advantageous to have kidneys that are programmed to avidly retain salt in a tropical climate, particularly in cultures with diets that are low in salt. However, in a temperate climate and with a high-salt diet, this genetic adaptation is a disadvantage and is considered an "abnormality in salt excretion" and a cause of hypertension.

People with this type of hypertension are considered to have salt-sensitive hypertension. A high-salt diet will elevate blood pressure and salt restriction will lower it. In this way, what was a genetic advantage can become what is considered a genetic defect in a different environment.

Salt-sensitive hypertension is determined both by how our kidneys handle salt and by how much salt we take in. Hypertension is salt sensitive in about 50 percent of African Americans who have hypertension but in only about 25 percent of whites with the condition. Older individuals are also more prone to salt-sensitive hypertension because of the age-related fall in the capacity of the kidneys to excrete salt.

Diuretics LOWER BLOOD PRESSURE by facilitating salt and fluid excretion by the kidneys. A diuretic is a drug of choice for people with salt-sensitive hypertension. The *calcium channel blockers,* which relax blood vessels by reducing the calcium concentration in the smooth muscle cells that line their walls, are also very effective in this type of hypertension.

Finally, in some people, salt-sensitive hypertension results from the failure of the renin–angiotensin system to turn off as it should in the presence of increased blood volume. In them, an ACE inhibitor, possibly in combination with a diuretic, is the logical treatment choice (see G. H. Williams, 1985).

Restriction of salt intake can lower blood pressure, sometimes even to normal, in people with salt-sensitive hypertension. You might even be able to avoid medication if you strictly limit your salt intake. The effect will be proportionate to the degree to which you reduce your intake of salt.

On the other hand, if you are not enthralled with a salt-free diet, or if salt restriction does not lower your blood pressure to normal, a diuretic is an important option for you. A pill a day of a diuretic does as good or better a job of lowering blood pressure than salt restriction does, and it works even if you do not watch your salt intake very closely. A diuretic is much more likely to lower your blood pressure to normal, although its use can cause unwanted effects such as gout or a reduced blood potassium level.

If you are taking a diuretic, I would caution against also severely restricting your salt intake, both because salt restriction adds only a little to the diuretic's blood pressure–lowering effect and because it increases the risk of dehydration. Even if you are not taking a diuretic, avoiding salt when your body craves and needs it—for example, after exercise on a hot, humid day—does more harm than good.

I would also like to convey a warning usually not mentioned by physicians or pharmacists: If you are taking a diuretic for hypertension and for any reason you are not eating, for example, because of the flu, skip the diuretic until you resume eating normally. Otherwise, you increase the risk of becoming dehydrated. This is a particular hazard in the elderly.

Like other drugs, diuretics should be used at the lowest dose possible. For example, I prescribe the commonly used diuretic, hydrochlorothiazide, at a dose of 12.5 or at most 25 milligrams per day. At these low doses, a potassium supplement usually is not necessary, although your blood potassium level should be checked periodically. If your potassium level is low, a potassium supplement or preferably a "potassium-sparing" diuretic, either alone or in combination with the diuretic you are taking, may be necessary. Sometimes, a low potassium level is a clue that excessive adrenal gland secretion of the hormone aldosterone is causing your hypertension. This is particularly likely if your potassium is low even without taking a diuretic. Your physician can tell you whether tests to look for this condition are warranted.

Treating Hypertension Caused by the Kidneys:
Targeting Volume or the Renin–Angiotensin System?
As illustrated in Figure 13.4, if your hypertension is driven by too much salt and volume, salt restriction or a diuretic will lower your blood pressure. If it is driven by the renin–angiotensin system, an ACE inhibitor or angiotensin antagonist will work better.

How can you tell which is the case and whether the effort to restrict salt intake is worthwhile for you? There are three ways. One is to attempt a trial of salt restriction to see whether your blood pressure falls. A second way is through demographics.

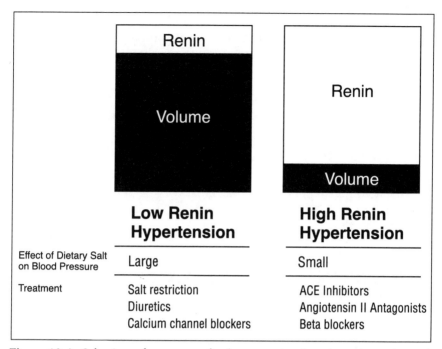

Figure 13.4. Selection of treatment for hypertension based on the reciprocal renin/volume relationship.

Hypertension in African Americans is more likely to fall in response to a diuretic than in response to an ACE inhibitor, and I therefore usually try a diuretic first. In white patients, either drug is equally likely to work. A third way is through measurement of the blood level of renin. People with salt- and volume-driven hypertension tend to have a low or medium renin level, whereas people with renin-driven hypertension tend to have a medium or high renin level.

Diuretics work best in people with low-renin hypertension, whereas ACE inhibitors, angiotensin antagonists, and beta blockers work best in people with medium- and high-renin hypertension. This is why it is wrong to automatically prescribe a diuretic as a first-choice drug for everyone with hypertension.

Salt restriction is also most likely to lower blood pressure in people with a low level of renin activity in the blood. As an approximate rule of thumb, approximately three of every four people with hypertension who have a low renin level will respond to salt restriction. Approximately two of four with a medium renin level and only one in four with a high renin level will respond.

This renin-based strategy improves the odds of selecting the right drug and helps in predicting whether restriction of salt intake will lower blood pressure. It is more helpful in guiding treatment in people with low- or high-renin hypertension. When the renin is in the medium range, as it is in more than half of people with hypertension, this strategy is less helpful. It also cannot tell us whether a person's hypertension is driven by the brain or by the kidney.

What Is Driving Your Hypertension: Brain or Kidney?

▶ Carla, a forty-five-year-old Ph.D. student, had had mild hypertension for several years. She told me she knew that the cause of her hypertension was that she was always frazzled and frequently faced deadlines. She had been prescribed different drugs, none of which had controlled her hypertension.

She seemed very much in touch with her feelings and was very aware of when she was tense. She was convinced that tension was the cause of her hypertension.

Based on my experience I suspected that her tenseness was not the cause of her hypertension. However, I went along with her assumption and prescribed a combination of an alpha blocker and a beta blocker to block the two limbs of the sympathoadrenal system. It had no effect on her blood pressure.

Switching to drugs directed at a genetic basis in the kidneys, with a combination of an ACE inhibitor and a diuretic, her blood pressure fell to normal. ◀

I see many patients who blame their hypertension on tension. Although worrying a lot doesn't feel good, it usually is not the cause of hypertension. Your blood pressure may go up at bad moments, but except in uncommon and extreme cases it does not stay up. I believe hypertension is more likely to occur in people who don't realize how tense they are than in people like Carla.

▶ John, forty-two, saw a colleague of mine for severe hypertension. Tests for a cause had been unrevealing, and treatment with an ACE inhibitor had been ineffective.

When my colleague sought my opinion, I asked him what John was like. He told me that John was a very nice guy, very relaxed, remarkably so, considering that he had recently been diagnosed with AIDS. He was coping beautifully and was not thrown by it.

To me this pointed almost paradoxically to hypertension driven by the brain. John's equanimity suggested that he was defended against feeling the severe distress related to his diagnosis. This distress could be expected to be far more severe than emotions related to a thesis deadline, yet its role was being ignored because John did not feel it or complain about it.

I suggested prescribing a combination of an alpha and beta blocker, even though John seemed calm. His systolic pressure fell to the 120s and has remained normal. ◀

The origin of John's hypertension was not evident from his appearance. It was evident from the same combination reported again and again in this book: the presence of a stress that could be expected to generate severe emotional distress in a person who claimed to feel perfectly calm.

We cannot judge someone to be calm because he claims to be, and even appears to be, calm. This is why the emotions you display don't reveal whether or not your hypertension is driven by the brain. Unless hidden emotions are considered, the origin of your hypertension is likely to remain obscure.

WHICH ORGAN DRIVES HYPERTENSION? Is it the brain, the seat of our emotions, or is it the kidneys? The answer is that in some people it is driven by the brain and in others it is driven by the kidneys. In still others, both are involved.

Whether hypertension originates in the brain or the kidney is not merely of theoretical interest. Drugs targeted at the sympathoadrenal system should work best in people whose hypertension originates in the brain; drugs targeted at the kidneys should work best in people whose hypertension originates in the kidneys.

It would seem very logical to select drugs this way. Why then does this rationale go unmentioned? It is amazing to me that no articles in medical journals discuss this very logical approach. Why is this approach unmentioned? Because no one knows how to identify in an individual whether the driving force of hypertension is the brain or the kidneys.

Neither renin measurement nor any other biochemical test can distinguish brain-driven from kidney-driven hypertension. Even without a biochemical test, it would seem easy to suggest that a nervous-appearing individual should be treated with a drug aimed at the brain, and a calm-appearing person should be treated with a drug aimed at the kidney. If the emotions we feel were the cause of hypertension, it would be simple to ask people how anxious, tense, or angry they were, or simply observe them and treat accordingly.

Unfortunately, this approach does not work. Carla's and John's cases illustrate why it does not. Carla's nervousness, apparent to her and perhaps to many around her, misleadingly suggested that her hypertension was emotion- and brain-driven. Emotions were not driving her hypertension, and therefore she did not respond to treatment directed at the sympathoadrenal system. Similarly, John's calmness, which seemed inappropriate in the face of his recent diagnosis of AIDS, misleadingly suggested that emotions were not related to his hypertension. Instead, almost counterintuitively, his *inappropriate* calmness provided the clue that his hypertension was emotion-driven.

These cases indicate yet again why selecting a treatment based on how people say they feel has not worked. The calm-appearing patient often is not calm inside and does not even know it. He fools himself and his physician, neither of whom would believe that his hypertension is driven by emotions. When instead we consider the role of hidden emotions, the treatment of hypertension begins to make more sense.

My experience suggests that hypertension mediated by the sympathetic nervous system is driven more by hidden emotions, and hypertension mediated by the kidneys is driven more by genetic factors. Treatment with drugs targeted at the sympathetic nervous system is more likely to be effective when hidden emotions are driving hypertension. Otherwise, treatment with drugs targeted at the kidneys is more likely to work, and identifying whether angiotensin or volume is driving your hypertension can further guide drug selection.

Finally, treatment directed at both mechanisms, sympathetic nervous system and kidneys, is sometimes necessary. In many people, both emotional and genetic factors underlie hypertension. In many people with longstanding hypertension, irreversible structural changes in blood vessels and damage to kidneys contribute to blood pressure elevation. Even if the original cause is eliminated, the blood pressure might remain elevated. At this stage the blood pressure usually cannot be brought down to normal without drugs such as ACE inhibitors and diuretics, which are directed at the effects of these structural abnormalities.

IN TRYING TO AVOID THE COMPLICATIONS of hypertension, the goal of treatment is to achieve a normal blood pressure with the least amount of medication necessary, combining the use of drug and nondrug therapies. I believe optimal treatment also involves selecting the therapies that match the cause of the hypertension.

We are best able to select the right drug or drugs if both the physical and emotional contributors are considered in the best spirit of mind–body medicine. This system will not work in every case, but the odds of finding the right drug are much better than the current system, which provides little rationale for selecting drugs.

CHAPTER 14

Healing, Medicine, and Society **14**

WESTERN MEDICINE HAS TRANSFORMED fatal illnesses into controllable conditions. It accomplishes miracles day in and day out—miracles that in the past would have been beyond our wildest hopes.

However, despite milestone after milestone in scientific progress, the cause or cure of many illnesses, such as hypertension, remains unknown. In some respects, in trying to understand why someone has hypertension, we have lost ground as we spend a fortune on diagnostic tests while ignoring the role of emotions, particularly those blocked from awareness.

Advocates of mind–body medicine traditionally suggest that the anger and anxiety we feel eventually lead to hypertension, and that relaxation techniques, biofeedback, and other measures to relieve emotional distress can cure it. Clearly these emotions are related to fluctuations in blood pressure and occasionally to hypertension, but studying and addressing them has largely failed to explain or alter the course of hypertension. Even the most severe forms of essential hypertension are as much a mystery today as they were decades ago. Even today, the leading hypertension experts in the world will throw their hands up when asked why someone has severe essential hypertension.

My main message in this book is to call for a paradigm shift in how we look at emotions and health. Given the long list of illnesses for which we have found neither the cause nor the cure, we can no longer ignore the importance of our hidden emotions.

WHAT I HAVE LEARNED from my patients is that it is the emotions we are hiding from ourselves, which we don't feel and often don't even know we harbor within us, that lead to hypertension. It is what conspicuously lacks an emotional impact that has more to do with hypertension than what is distressing to us.

These emotions might originate from abuse during childhood, whose effects we had to hide from ourselves. Or they might originate from trauma that we suffered at any age. Or they might be the emotions that day after day, without knowing it, we hide from ourselves because hiding them is the only way we know.

The importance of the link between hidden emotions and hypertension is not limited to the rare patient. It is relevant to millions of people taking medication for high blood pressure. It can open up a new approach to treatment based on emotional healing.

Many people consider the suggestion of an emotional basis for physical illness as an accusation of emotional weakness or illness. It was hard for me to learn how to convey to patients that there is an emotional basis for hypertension, but it is not the result of an emotional weakness or infirmity. On the contrary, people do emotionally what they needed to do to survive.

Hiding emotions is usually a way of survival rather than a sign of psychopathology; that is why we were born with the capacity to hide them. It is the person who could not hide emotions when it was necessary who is more likely to be troubled emotionally. Our ability to hide what we needed to hide is a gift. To acknowledge that we harbor such emotions is not an admission of emotional illness but is a step to reclaim our wholeness.

The Need to Return to Clinical Observations

The purported role in hypertension of the emotions we feel, and the concepts of anger and stress management, have not been ignored. The National Institutes of Health has funded many hundreds of studies, performed not by the skeptical antipsychology medical establishment but by research psychologists who believe in the mind–body connection. The more scientifically controlled the studies, the less the observed relationship they have shown between the emotions we feel and hypertension, and the less the observed benefit of interventions aimed at them. These interventions are ignored by the medical establishment not for lack of study or attention but because the inconsistency of their results has taught us that addressing those emotions plays a limited role in treating hypertension.

The scientific method cannot be applied easily in studying hidden emotions. We cannot measure the emotions we do not feel. Yet it would be foolish to discount the role of what we cannot measure in an era when so many illnesses and physical symptoms are still begging for an explanation.

Questionnaires that are useful in studying the emotions we feel have much less value in studying our hidden emotions. A researcher who does not even meet the people being studied, but who merely hands them a questionnaire, cannot appreciate the role of emotions that lie beneath the surface. If we are to understand hypertension, research must return to people rather than solely focusing on measurements and statistics.

Clinical observations have been the driving force in solving many medical mysteries. They complement laboratory research and fill in the gap of what research does not, and perhaps cannot, explain. The role of hidden emotions in hypertension became apparent to me only through repeated clinical observations, through listening to patients and their stories. It became apparent through observing the disappearance of hypertension after hidden emotions were brought into awareness in the context of the doctor–patient relationship. I have observed phenomena that cannot occur in the controlled circumstances of a laboratory or according to a study timetable. Illuminating cases like Martha's in Chapter 5, whose shift in awareness occurred six years after I began treating her, cannot be observed in a laboratory.

Confirmation of such observations in large studies is desirable but will be difficult and expensive and will require many years. It will require considerable support from those who control distribution of research funding.

In the meantime, I hope that the clinical observations I have reported, the sense they can make of hypertension and other physical disorders that have remained unexplained, and the existing scientific evidence that already backs them up, will stimulate interest in the long-neglected role of our hidden emotions in health. I hope they will provoke awareness among patients, physicians, and researchers, and help promote a new era in uniting the treatment of body and mind.

Making Sense of Hypertension and Other Illnesses

The origin of many prominent medical illnesses still defies explanation by the biological model of Western medicine. Paying attention to the emotions we have hidden can provide answers that decades of medical research have not provided. It can make sense of hypertension and of many other illnesses and symptoms that until now have made no sense to us.

Too often when a person has unexplained physical symptoms and reports no particular emotional distress, endless medical testing has remained the path followed almost exclusively. When testing fails to find a cause, I believe it is a disservice to people to fail to consider an origin in emotions they would not suspect are affecting them. Most physicians and patients are not accustomed to thinking about physical symptoms or illness in this way. Yet this does not conflict with the Western approach to treatment. It complements it. It can take over where Western medicine leaves off, where Western medicine acknowledges that it can offer neither understanding nor cure, only treatment to suppress symptoms or reduce complications.

The challenge of understanding the mind–body link of hypertension and other conditions involves understanding when emotions lie at their heart and also when they do not. Hidden emotions are not always the cause of hypertension. Genetics and lifestyle factors also govern blood pressure to a large extent. It is a disservice to mind–body medicine, and reduces its credibility, when we blame all of hypertension or other conditions on emotions. Instead, as I've discussed in Chapter 10, it is important to look at people individually and to try to identify those in whom emotions are involved and those in whom they are not.

The Rewards of Seeking a Healing Process

A path of awareness is not an option for some people. Fortunately, for many others it is. Even though we don't realize it, we often have the strength to face our hidden emotions if we choose to do so. The pleasant surprise to me is that many of my patients do choose this path. It is not that they had been unable to do so previously. It is simply that it had never before occurred to them to address emotions they did not know they were concealing within them.

Getting in touch with the emotions hidden within us can heal illness and can also transform our lives. Healing is not just removal of illness. It is removal of the barriers keeping us from being fully who we were meant to be. Theresa and Martha, whose stories were discussed in Chapter 5, did not just relieve their hypertension. They also realized how they had accepted being victimized. They changed their relationships, but only after they had gained this awareness.

In my experience, patients who gained awareness of their estrangement from a part of themselves experienced a rapid and persisting improvement in hypertension and other conditions. They defy the conventional wisdom that a long time is needed before any healing awareness can take place. In addition, once a shift has occurred, once a person realizes the impact of what she has hidden away and her ability to embrace her emotions, she is better prepared to begin to embrace other emotions she previously dared not face. Thus, the initial change, even if limited, can lead to more change over time and to true emotional healing.

Many, however, strongly resist awareness of hidden emotions. Ironically, the more we are hiding, the less likely we are to be aware that we are doing so and the more insistent we are that we have nothing to hide. The more our health is affected by what we are hiding, the more likely we are to insist that emotions are not involved in our illness. This is the paradox and the true challenge of the mind–body connection.

Achieving awareness of our hidden emotions can be difficult and painful. We have resisted feeling these emotions for good reason. We are not eager to seek that which we have hidden away. The healing process requires considerable commitment, time, and support. I encounter many patients who do not choose this road. However, I encounter many others who do.

The Crisis of Connectedness in Our Evolving Society

Underlying the barrier to much of our emotions is the isolation in which we hold them. The effects of that isolation on our physical health are only beginning to be told.

Although advances in technology may advance our ability to decipher mysteries at a microscopic and molecular level, they are less able to advance our understanding of emotional and spiritual relatedness and wholeness. However, that doesn't make emotional relatedness an invalid or irrelevant concept. Our connectedness with each other is a powerful weapon against mental and physical illness, but we do little to foster it. Although we are born with an innate drive for connectedness, if we are not exposed to it we do not develop our capacity for it and we lose sight of that drive. Eventually, we do not even realize it is missing.

The observation most striking to me is how often emotional connectedness is absent in the lives of patients I talk to, and how often they do not even realize it. Even if surrounded by people, they handle their most difficult emotions alone, not knowing there is any other way. They do not confide their distress, even when surrounded by people who love them. They do not know what it feels like. Supplying connectedness to them does not change this. Raising awareness of its absence is needed first.

Many factors are conspiring to create a society with less and less connectedness. Families are smaller and geographically separated. The nuclear family is fractured in many homes, whether by divorce or friction. The close extended family is the exception more than the rule. The intimate community is harder to maintain amid urban congestion. The glut of work, chores, and diversions enables us to keep busy every minute of every day, and to be strangers to our emotions, to ourselves, and to those around us. Despite our technological progress, or perhaps because of it, we are living in a different world and we are paying a price for it.

As the nuclear family declines, more and more children are growing up without the experience of connectedness. Perhaps one way to break this growing grip of isolation would be to create groups in which children could experience and learn the safety and comfort of confiding their emotions. The cost-benefit potential to society could be staggering.

Although we are battling many factors that promote emotional isolation, we also live in an era in which an emotional transformation is highly possible. We have reduced famine and hunger in many parts of the world. We live longer and presumably accumulate more wisdom. We have the technology and freedom to communicate thoughts and ideas to everyone. The field of psychology complements religion in teaching us about our barriers to relatedness. We are beginning to acknowledge and tackle abuse of children and the consequences of that abuse. More than ever, we are in a position to begin to open ourselves up emotionally.

More and more we are dissatisfied with the status quo. We know that the fruits of technology have not brought us emotional peace. We know hedonistic pleasures leave us dissatisfied, even if it takes a while to find that out. The publication and purchases of book after book written as guides for a spiritual search testify to the increasing realization of our need to heal within.

The seeds are in place to begin a transformation in our relatedness and connectedness. Such change will also go far in reducing the physical ailments that result from our isolation.

My View as a Physician

A physician is in a position to listen to the concerns of his or her patients, and, merely by doing so, to provide comfort. People often feel more free to mention things to their physician than to others.

However, there are major barriers that keep patients from confiding in the context of this relationship. Aside from the possible lack of time, interest, or skill on the part of the physician, the distressful emotions that are perhaps the most relevant to health go unmentioned because patients and physicians are equally unaware of them. Patient and doctor willingly pursue test after test to discover the cause of unexplained and unexplainable physical illness, while never digging below the surface, to touch on the emotions the patient does not, and often cannot, report.

I have found that many patients with comfortable lives have a past history of emotional trials that I never would have suspected—trials that they have not discussed with anyone. I find I am often the first person to talk with them about events that irreversibly changed their lives years or even decades ago.

THE STORIES I HAVE TOLD are not a collection of highly unusual cases. They are stories of patients from a single medical practice in a single city. I suspect that such observations are not reported more widely for one very simple reason: Physicians do not inquire about unfelt emotions or about emotions hidden long ago and not discussed for decades. I believe the cases I describe in this book are unique in hypertension literature only because I look for what is hidden.

In an ideal world, the basis in hidden emotions underlying hypertension and other illnesses could be uncovered in the setting of the doctor–patient relationship. Obviously, for many reasons this is unlikely to happen, which is why I wrote this book for people with hypertension. The cycle of endless physical symptoms and unexplained physical illnesses such as hypertension can be interrupted only if people are willing to consider a different view of them. In the end, in many ways, we are each responsible for our own health.

I HOPE THE STORIES I HAVE TOLD will stimulate you to think about the emotions you might be hiding. This is an exercise you might have never performed, having long ago decided that past events have no lingering effects and that emotions cannot be affecting you if you do not feel upset.

I urge you to reflect on your life, on the difficult times, past or present, even though you would rather ignore them. If you have stabilized your life, you are in a better position to do so, and to literally console yourself for what you have had to endure and could only endure by ceasing to feel. I urge you to talk with someone who is close to you, who you know will respect your emotions, whatever they are, and who will have the patience to listen to your story with respect.

If you are concerned about taking care of everyone but yourself, consider the price you are paying. You need not assume that your needs don't matter or that your life can never change.

Healing physically is inseparable from healing emotionally from the hurt and isolation we refuse to see or acknowledge. We focus on the smaller external stresses instead of bringing to an end our alienation from ourselves. However, when we shift and acknowledge our barrier to awareness, we can create major changes in our life and health.

Our past is the foundation of who we are today, both good and bad. It has both hurt us and helped us. It has motivated us to seek the security we once lacked and to excel. It has given us a purpose that we otherwise might not have had in our work and in how we parent our children. For these reasons, we can honor the suffering rather than isolate it from our awareness.

Our emotions are a valuable guide to us. Our emotional sensors alert us when things are not right. If we are not in touch with them, we will not have the motivation to seek the changes we need in our lives and relationships. We cannot learn new ways of behavior or of communication if we do not feel upset with the way things are. Our distress is the impetus that moves us to change. We pay a price when we try to ignore it.

WE WERE CREATED with the capacity to block our awareness when we need to and to regain that awareness when it is time to heal. When we realize that we have this capacity, we can open a new avenue to health and wholeness. When we realize our barriers are within us, no one can stop us from regaining the unity that resides inside us, that is ours to take.

Antihypertensive Drugs

I. Drugs directed primarily at the brain and sympathoadrenal system (see Chapter 13 for further description)

A. *Beta adrenergic blockers*

Generic Names	Popular Brand Names
acebutolol	Sectral
atenolol	Tenormin
betaxolol	Kerlone
bisoprolol	Zebeta
metoprolol	Lopressor, Toprol
nadolol	Corgard
penbutolol	Levatol
pindolol	Visken
propranolol	Inderal
timolol	Blocadren

B. *Alpha adrenergic blockers*

Generic Names	Popular Brand Names
doxazosin	Cardura
prazosin	Minipress
terazosin	Hytrin

C. *Combined alpha/beta blockers*

Generic Names	Popular Brand Names
carvedilol	Coreg
labetolol	Trandate, Normodyne

D. *Central alpha agonists*

Generic Names	Popular Brand Names
clonidine	Catapres, Catapres patch
guanabenz	Wytensin
guanfacine	Tenex
methyldopa	Aldomet

E. *Peripheral-acting adrenergic inhibitors*

Generic Names	Popular Brand Names
guanadrel	Hylorel
guanethidine	Ismelin
reserpine	Serpasil

II. Drugs directed primarily at the kidney

A. *Angiotensin-converting enzyme inhibitors (ACE inhibitors)*

Generic Names	Popular Brand Names
benazapril	Lotensin
captopril	Capoten
enalapril	Vasotec
fosinopril	Monopril
lisinopril	Prinivil, Zestril
moexipril	Univasc
quinapril	Accupril
ramipril	Altace
trandolapril	Mavik

B. *Diuretics*

Generic Names	Popular Brand Names

1. *Thiazides and related agents*

chlorthalidone	Hygroton
chlorothiazide	Diuril
hydrochlorothiazide	Hydrodiuril
indapamide	Lozol
metolazone	Zaroxalyn

2. *Loop diuretics*

bumetanide	Bumex
ethacrynic acid	Edecrin
furosemide	Lasix
torsemide	Demedex

3. *Potassium-sparing diuretics*

amiloride	Midamor
spironolactone	Aldactone
triamterene	Dyrenium

4. *Combined thiazide/potassium-sparing diuretics*

hydrochlorothiazide/amiloride	Moduretic
hydrochlorothiazide/spironolactone	Aldactazide
hydrochlorothiazide/triamterene	Dyazide, Maxzide

C. *Angiotensin-II receptor antagonists*

Generic Names	*Popular Brand Names*
irbesartan	Avapro
losartan	Cozaar
valsartan	Diovan

III. Blood vessel dilators that are not specifically directed at the brain or kidney

A. *Calcium channel blockers*

Generic Names	*Popular Brand Names*

1. *Nondihydropyridine*

diltiazem	Cardizem, Tiazac
verapamil	Calan, Isoptin, Verelan, Covera

2. *Dihydropyridine*

amlodipine	Norvasc
felodipine	Plendil
isradipine	Dynacirc
nicardipine	Cardene
nifedipine	Procardia, Adalat
nisoldipine	Sular

B. *Direct vasodilators*

Generic Names	*Popular Brand Names*
hydralazine	Apresoline
minoxidil	Loniten

IV. Combination drugs

A. *Beta blocker—diuretic*
Corzide (nadolol with bendroflumethiazide)
Inderide (propranolol with hydrochlorothiazide)
Lopressor HCT (metoprolol with hydrochlorothiazide)
Tenoretic (atenolol with chlorthalidone)
Timolide (timolol with hydrochlorothiazide)
Ziac (bisoprolol with hydrochlorothiazide)

B. *ACE inhibitor—diuretic*
Capozide (captopril with hydrochlorothiazide)
Lotensin HCT (benazepril with hydrochlorothiazide)
Prinizide, Zestoretic (lisinopril with hydrochlorothiazide)
Vaseretic (enalapril with hydrochlorothiazide)

C. *Angiotensin antagonist with diuretic*
Hyzaar (losartan with hydrochlorothiazide)

D. *ACE inhibitor—calcium channel blocker*
Lexxel (enalapril with felodipine)
Lotrel (benazepril with amlodipine)
Tarka (trandolapril with verapamil)
Teczem (enalapril with diltiazem)

E. *Others*
Combipres (clonidine with chlorthalidone)
Minizide (prazosin with polythiazide)

Bibliography

Alexander CN, Schneider RH, Staggers F, et al. Trial of stress reduction for hypertension in older African Americans. II Sex and risk subgroup analysis. *Hypertension* 28: 228, 1996.

Allander PS, Cutler JA, Follmann D, et al. Dietary calcium and blood pressure: a meta-analysis of randomized clinical trials. *Annals of Internal Medicine* 124: 825, 1996.

Amigo I, Cuesta V, Fernandez A, et al. The effect of verbal instructions on blood pressure measurement. *Journal of Hypertension* 11: 293, 1993.

Anderson GH, Blakeman N, Streeten DH. The effect of age on prevalence of secondary forms of hypertension in 4429 consecutively referred patients. *Journal of Hypertension* 12: 609, 1994.

Appel LJ, Moore TJ, Obarzanek E, et al. A clinical trial of dietary patterns on blood pressure. *New England Journal of Medicine* 336: 1117, 1997.

Asendorpf JB, Scherer KR. The discrepant repressor: differentiation between low anxiety, high anxiety, and repression of anxiety by autonomic-facial-verbal patterns of behavior. *Journal of Personality and Social Research* 45: 1334, 1983.

Attwood S, Bird R, Burch K, et al. Within-patient correlation between the antihypertensive effects of atenolol, lisinopril and nifedipine. *Journal of Hypertension* 12: 1053, 1994.

Australian Therapeutic Trial in Mild Hypertension. *Lancet* 1: 1261, 1980.

Benson H. *The Relaxation Response.* New York: William Morrow and Co., Inc., 1975.

Benson H. Systemic hypertension and the relaxation response. *New England Journal of Medicine* 296: 1152, 1977.

Berkman LF, Leo-Summers L, Horwitz RI. Emotional support and survival after myocardial infarction. A prospective, population-based study of the elderly. *Annals of Internal Medicine* 117: 1003, 1992.

Bettelheim B. Afterword to C. Vegh, *I Didn't Say Goodbye*, trans. R Schwartz. New York: EP Dutton, 1984, p. 166.

Borhani NO, Borkman TS. *The Alameda County Blood Pressure Study.* Berkeley, California: State of California Department of Public Health, 1968.

Bradshaw J. Homecoming. Reclaiming and Championing Your Inner Child. New York: Bantam Books, 1990.

Burt VL, Whelton P, Roccella EJ, et al. Prevalence of hypertension in the U.S. adult population. Results from the third National Health and Nutrition examination survey, 1988–1991. *Hypertension* 25: 305, 1995.

Cottier C, Perini C, Rauchfleisch U. Personality traits and hypertension: an overview. In *Handbook of Hypertension,* volume 9: *Behavioral Factors in Hypertension,* S Julius and DR Bassett, editors. Amsterdam: Elsevier Science Publishers B.V., 1987, pp. 123–140.

Cottington EM, Brock BM, House JS, et al. Psychosocial factors and blood pressure in the Michigan Statewide blood pressure survey. *American Journal of Epidemiology* 121: 515, 1985.

Crowne DP, Marlowe D. A new scale of social desirability independent of psychopathology. *Journal of Consulting Psychology* 24: 349, 1960.

Cutler JA, Follmann D, Elliott P, et al. An overview of randomized trials of sodium reduction and blood pressure. *Hypertension* 17 (supplement I): I-27, 1991.

Dafter RE. Why "negative" emotions can sometimes be positive: The spectrum model of emotions and their role in mind–body healing. *Advances* 12: 6, 1996.

Depression Guideline Panel. *Depression in Primary Care,* volume 1: *Detection and Diagnosis* (Clinical Practice Guideline No. 5). Rockville, Maryland: Department of Health and Human Services, 1993. AHCPR publication No. 93-0550.

Drossman DA, Leserman J, Nachman G, et al. Sexual and physical abuse in women with functional or organic gastrointestinal disorders. *Annals of Internal Medicine* 113: 828, 1990.

Eisenberg DM, Delbanco TL, Berkey CS. Cognitive behavioral techniques for hypertension: Are they effective? *Annals of Internal Medicine* 118: 964, 1993.

Esler M. Biochemical evidence for sympathetic overactivity in human hypertension. In *Handbook of Hypertension,* volume 9: *Behavioral Factors in Hypertension,* S Julius and DR Bassett, editors. Amsterdam: Elsevier Science Publishers B.V., 1987, pp. 75–94.

Fagard RH. The role of exercise in blood pressure control: supportive evidence. *Journal of Hypertension* 13: 1223, 1995.

Feinblatt A, Meighan D. Short-term group psychotherapy for chronic pain. *Psychosomatic Medicine* 60: 119, 1998.

Floras JS, Hara K. Sympathoneural and haemodynamic characteristics of young subjects with mild essential hypertension. *Journal of Hypertension* 11: 647–655, 1993.

Freud S. *Repression,* J Strachey, editor, *The Standard Edition of the Complete Works of Sigmund Freud,* volume 14, 1915/1957, pp. 146–158.

Goldstein DS. *Stress, Catecholamines and Cardiovascular Disease.* New York: Oxford University Press, 1995.

Grassi G. Editor's corner: evaluating sympathetic and haemodynamic responses to mental stressors: hankering or achievement? *Journal of Hypertension* 14: 1155, 1996.

Gross J. Emotional expression in cancer onset and progression. *Social Science and Medicine* 28: 1239, 1989.

Haehn K-D. Psychological approaches to improve patient compliance. *Journal of Hypertension* 3 (supplement 1): 61, 1985.

Hunyor SN, Henderson RJ. The role of stress management in blood pressure control: why the promissory note has failed to deliver. *Journal of Hypertension* 14: 413, 1996.

Jacob RG, Shapiro AP, O'Hara P. Relaxation therapy for hypertension: setting-specific effects. *Psychosomatic Medicine* 54: 87, 1992.

James GD, Yee LS, Harshfield GA, et al. The influence of happiness, anger and anxiety on the blood pressure of borderline hypertensives. *Psychosomatic Medicine* 48: 502, 1986.

Johnston DW, Gold A, Kentish J, et al. Effect of stress management on blood pressure in mild primary hypertension. *British Medical Journal* 306: 963, 1993.

Joint National Committee on Prevention, Detection, Evaluation and Treatment of High Blood Pressure: Fifth Report: *Archives of Internal Medicine* 153: 154, 1993. Sixth Report: *Archives of Internal Medicine* 157: 2413, 1997.

Jorgensen RS, Johnson BT, Kolodziej ME, et al. Elevated blood pressure and personality: a meta-analytic review. *Psychological Bulletin* 120: 293, 1996.

Joseph R. *The Right Brain and the Unconscious: Discovering the Stranger Within.* New York: Plenum, 1992.

Julius S. Sympathetic hyperactivity and coronary risk in hypertension. *Hypertension* 21: 886, 1993.

Julius S, Schork MA. Borderline hypertension: a critical review. *Journal of Chronic Diseases* 23: 723, 1971.

Jung CG, *The Undiscovered Self,* in Bollingen Series XX, *The Collected Works of C. G. Jung,* volume 10, H Read, M Fordham, and G Adler, editors. New York: Bollingen Foundation, 1964, p. 292.

Kahn HA, Medalie JH, Neufeld HN, et al. The incidence of hypertension and associated factors: the Israeli Ischemic Heart Disease Study. *American Heart Journal* 84: 171, 1972.

Kaplan NM. *Clinical Hypertension,* 6th Edition. Baltimore: Williams and Wilkins, 1994, pp. 55–56.

Karasu TB. The psychotherapies: benefits and limitations. *American Journal of Psychotherapy* 40: 324, 1986.

Kelley G, McClellan P. Antihypertensive effects of aerobic exercise: a brief meta-analytic review of randomized controlled trials. *American Journal of Hypertension* 7: 115, 1994.

King AC, Taylor CB, Albright CA, et al. The relationship between repressive and defensive coping styles and blood pressure responses in healthy, middle-aged men and women. *Journal of Psychosomatic Research* 34: 461, 1990.

Kobasa SC, Puccetti MC. Personal and social resources in stress resistance. *Journal of Personality and Social Psychology* 45: 839, 1983.

Krantz DS, Manuck SB. Acute psychophysiologic reaction and risk of cardiovascular disease: a review and methodology critique. *Psychological Bulletin* 96: 435, 1984.

Krieger N, Sidney S. Racial discrimination and blood pressure: the CARDIA study of young black and white adults. *American Journal of Public Health* 86: 1370, 1996.

Kroenke K, Mangelsdorff AD. Common symptoms in ambulatory care: incidence, evaluation, therapy and outcome. *American Journal of Medicine* 86: 262, 1989.

Laragh JH. Issues, goals and guidelines in selecting first-line therapy for hypertension. *Hypertension* 13 (suppl. 5): S103, 1989.

Lazerus RS. The costs and benefits of denial. In *The Denial of Stress,* S Bresnitz, editor. New York: International University Press, 1983, pp. 1–33.

Light KC. Cardiovascular responses to effortful coping: implications for the role of stress in hypertension development. *Psychophysiology* 18: 216, 1981.

Linden W, Feuerstein M. Essential hypertension and social coping behavior: experimental findings. *Journal of Human Stress* 9: 22, 1983.

Lindquist TL, Beilin LJ, Knuiman MW. Influence of lifestyle, coping and job stress on blood pressure in men and women. *Hypertension* 29: 1, 1997.

Lynch JJ. *The Language of the Heart. The Human Body in Dialogue.* New York: Basic Books, 1985, pp. 134–136.

MacMillan HL, Fleming JE, Trocme N, et al. Prevalence of child physical and sexual abuse in the community. Results from the Ontario Health Supplement. *Journal of the American Medical Association* 278: 131, 1997.

Mann SJ. Severe paroxysmal hypertension. An autonomic syndrome and its relationship to repressed emotions. *Psychosomatics* 37: 444, 1996.

Mann SJ, Delon M. Improved hypertension control after disclosure of decades-old trauma. *Psychosomatic Medicine* 57: 501, 1995.

Mann SJ, James GD. Repressive coping and obesity as co-factors in the etiology of essential hypertension. *American Journal of Hypertension* 9: 97A, 1996.

Mann SJ, James GD. Defensiveness and essential hypertension. *Journal of Psychosomatic Research* 45: 139, 1998.

Mann, SJ. Severe paroxysmal hypertension (pseudopheochromocytoma): understanding the cause and treatment. *Archives of Internal Medicine* (in press).

Matthews DA, Suchman AL, Branch WT Jr. Making "connexions": enhancing the therapeutic potential of patient-clinician relationships. *Annals of Internal Medicine* 118: 973, 1993.

McMahon SW, Blacket RB, McDonald GJ, et al. Obesity, alcohol consumption and blood pressure in Australian men and women. The National Heart Foundation of Australia Risk Factor Prevention Study. *Journal of Hypertension* 2: 85, 1984.

Medical Research Council Working Party (MRC). Trial of treatment of mild hypertension: principal results. *British Medical Journal* 291: 97, 1985.

Mellinger GD, Balter MB, Uhlenhuth EH. Insomnia and its treatment: prevalence and correlates. *Archives of General Psychiatry* 42: 225, 1985.

Menard J. Improving hypertension treatment. Where should we put our efforts: new drugs, new concepts or new management? *American Journal of Hypertension* 5 (supplement): 252S, 1992.

Meyer E, Derogates LR, Miller M, et al. Hypertension and psychological distress. *Psychosomatics* 19: 160, 1978.

Monk M. Psychological status and hypertension. *American Journal of Epidemiology* 112: 200, 1980.

Montfrans GA, Karemaker JM, Wieling W, et al. Relaxation therapy and continuous ambulatory blood pressure in mild hypertension: a controlled study. *British Medical Journal* 300: 1368, 1990.

Morris MC, Sacks F, Rosner B. Does fish oil lower blood pressure? A meta-analysis of controlled trials. *Circulation* 88: 523, 1993.

Norris FH. Epidemiology of trauma: frequency and impact of different potentially traumatic events on different demographic groups. *Journal of Consulting and Clinical Psychology* 60: 409, 1992.

Panfilov VV, Reid JL. Brain and autonomic mechanisms in hypertension. *Journal of Hypertension* 12: 337–343, 1994.

Parati G, Pomidossi G, Casadei R, et al. Comparison of the cardiovascular effects of different laboratory stressors and their relationship to blood pressure variability. *Journal of Hypertension* 6: 481, 1988.

Peled-Ney R, Silverberg DS, Rosenfeld JB. A controlled study of group therapy in essential hypertension. *Israeli Journal of Medical Science* 20: 12, 1984.

Pelligrine RJ. Repression-sensitization and perceived severity of presenting problem of four hundred and forty-four counseling center clients. *Journal of Counseling Psychology* 18: 332, 1971.

Pickering TG, Gerin W. Cardiovascular reactivity in the laboratory and the role of behavioral factors in hypertension: a critical review. *Annals of Behavioral Medicine* 12: 3, 1990.

Pickering TG, James GD, Boddie C, et al. How common is white coat hypertension? *Journal of the American Medical Association* 259: 225, 1988.

Pogue, VA, Ellis C, Michel J, et al. New staging system of the Fifth Joint National Committee Report on the Detection, Evaluation and Treatment of High Blood Pressure (JNC V) alters assessment and severity of treatment of hypertension. *Hypertension* 28: 713, 1996.

Puddey IB, Beilin LJ, Vandongen R. Regular alcohol use raises blood pressure in treated hypertensive subjects. A randomized controlled trial. *Lancet* 1: 647, 1987.

Ross ED, Homan RW, Buck R. Differential hemispheric lateralization of primary and social emotions. Implications for developing a comprehensive neurology for emotions, repression, and the subconscious. *Neuropsychiatry, Neuropsychology and Behavioral Neurology* 7: 1, 1994.

Rostrup M, Kjeldsen SE, Eide IK. Awareness of hypertension increases blood pressure and sympathetic responses to cold pressor test. *American Journal of Hypertension* 3: 912, 1990.

Ruberman W, Weinblatt E, Goldberg JD. Psychosocial influences on mortality after myocardial infarction. *New England Journal of Medicine* 311: 552, 1984.

Ruddy MC, Bialy GB, Malka ES, et al. The relationship of plasma renin activity to clinic and ambulatory blood pressure in elderly people with isolated systolic hypertension. *Journal of Hypertension* 6 (supplement 4): S412, 1988.

Russek LG, Schwartz GE. Perceptions of parental caring predict health status in midlife: a 35-year follow-up of the Harvard Mastery of Stress Study. *Psychosomatic Medicine* 59: 144, 1997.

Sarno J. *Healing Back Pain. The Mind–Body Connection.* New York: Warner Books, 1991.

Schotte DE, Stunkard AJ. The effects of weight reduction on blood pressure in 301 obese subjects. *Archives of Internal Medicine* 150: 1701, 1990.

Shapiro F, Silk Forrest M. *EMDR. The Breakthrough Therapy for Overcoming Anxiety, Stress, and Trauma.* New York: Basic Books, 1997.

Shedler J, Mayman M, Manis M. The illusion of mental health. *American Psychologist* 48: 1117, 1993.

Silagy CA, Neil HAW. A meta-analysis of the effect of garlic on blood pressure. *Journal of Hypertension* 12: 463, 1994.

Silverberg DS, Oksenberg A, Iaina A. Sleep-related breathing disorders are common contributing factors to the production of essential hypertension but are neglected, underdiagnosed and undertreated. *American Journal of Hypertension* 10: 1319, 1997.

Sommers-Flanagan J, Greenberg RP. Psychosocial variables and hypertension: a new look at an old controversy. *Journal of Nervous and Mental Diseases* 177: 15, 1989.

Spiegel D, Bloom JR, Kraemer HC, et al. Effect of psychosocial treatment on survival of patients with metastatic breast cancer. *Lancet* 2: 888, 1989.

Stamler R, Stamler J, Riedlinger WF, et al. Weight and blood pressure findings in hypertension screening of one million Americans. *Journal of the American Medical Association* 240: 1607, 1978.

Steiner H. Repressive adaptation and family environment. *Acta Paedopsychiatrica* 55: 121, 1992.

Stewart WF, Schechter A, Rasmussen BK. Migraine prevalence: a review of population-based studies. *Neurology* 44 (supplement 4): S17, 1994.

Strickland BR, Crowne DP. Need for approval and the premature termination of psychotherapy. *Journal of Consulting Psychology* 27: 95, 1963.

Sullivan J, Hanson P, Rahko PS, et al. Continuous measurement of left ventricular performance during and after maximal isometric deadlift exercise. *Circulation* 85: 1406, 1992.

Suls J, Wan CK, Costa PT Jr. Relationship of trait anger to resting blood pressure: a meta-analysis. *Health Psychology* 14: 444, 1995.

Thelen MK. Repression-sensitization: its relation to adjustment and seeking psychotherapy among college students. *Journal of Consulting Psychology* 33: 161, 1969.

Toner BB, Koyama E, Garfinkle PE, et al. Social desirability and Irritable Bowel Syndrome. *International Journal of Psychiatry in Medicine* 22: 99, 1992.

Trials of Hypertension Prevention Collaborative Research Group. The effects of nonpharmacologic interventions on blood pressure of persons with high normal levels: results of the Trials of Hypertension Prevention, Phase I. *Journal of the American Medical Association* 267: 1213, 1992.

Van der Kolk BA, McFarlane AC, Weisaeth L, editors. *Traumatic Stress. The Effects of Overwhelming Experience on Mind, Body and Spirit.* New York: Guilford Press, 1996, p. 548.

Wagner PJ, Mongan P, Hendrick LK, et al. Experience of abuse in primary care patients: racial and rural differences. *Archives of Family Medicine* 4: 956, 1995.

Ward R. Familial aggregation and genetic epidemiology of blood pressure. In *Hypertension: Pathophysiology, Diagnosis and Management,* 2nd edition, JH Laragh and BM Brenner, editors. New York: Raven Press, 1995, pp. 67–88.

Warrenberg S, Levine J, Schwartz GE, et al. Defensive coping and blood pressure reactivity in medical patients. *Journal of Behavioral Medicine* 12: 407, 1989.

Weder AB, Julius S. Behavior, blood pressure variability and hypertension. *Psychosomatic Medicine* 47: 406, 1985.

Weil A. *Spontaneous Healing.* New York: Random House, 1995.

Weinberger DA, Davidson MN. Styles of inhibiting emotional expression: distinguishing repressive coping from impression management. *Journal of Personality* 62: 587, 1994.

Weinberger DA, Schwartz GE, Davidson RJ. Low-anxious, high-anxious and repressive coping styles: psychometric patterns and behavioral and physiological responses to stress. *Journal of Abnormal Psychology* 88: 369, 1979.

Weiner H, Sapira JD. Hypertension: a challenge to behavioral research. In *Handbook of Hypertension,* volume 9: *Behavioral Factors in Hypertension,* S Julius and DR Bassett, editors. Amsterdam: Elsevier Science Publishers B.V., 1987, pp. 259–284.

Wennerholm MA, Zarle TH. Internal-external control, defensiveness and anxiety in hypertensive patients. *Journal of Clinical Psychology* 32: 644, 1976.

Whitfield CL. *Memory and Abuse. Remembering and Healing the Effects of Trauma.* Deerfield, Florida: Health Communications, Inc., 1995.

Wiley RL, Dunn CL, Cox RH, et al. Isometric exercise training lowers resting blood pressure. *Medicine and Science in Sports and Exercise* 24: 749, 1992.

Williams GH, Hollenberg NK. Non-modulating essential hypertension: a subset particularly responsive to converting enzyme inhibitors. *Journal of Hypertension* 3 (suppl. 2): S817, 1985.

Winkleby MA, Raglano DR, Syme SL. Self-reported stressors and hypertension: evidence of an inverse association. *American Journal of Epidemiology* 127: 124, 1988.

Wolf S, Pfeiffer JB, Ripley HS, et al. Hypertension as a reaction pattern to stress: summary of experimental data on variations in blood pressure and renal blood flow. *Annals of Internal Medicine* 29: 1056, 1948.

Zinn W. The empathic physician. *Archives of Internal Medicine* 153: 306, 1993.

Index

ACE inhibitor (angiotensin-converting enzyme inhibitor), 152, 194, 201, 203, 204, 205–6, 207, 208, 209, 213
adrenaline, 121, 137, 196, 197, 198, 202, 203, 205
adrenal limb, 196, 197, 198, 204, 208
African Americans, 88, 89, 190, 207, 208
Alameda County Blood Pressure Study, 88
alcohol consumption, 15, 191
Aldomet (methyldopa), 127
aldosterone, 137, 196, 204, 208
alerting reaction, 21–22, 23, 25, 28
Alexander, Charles, 38, 177
Allander, P. Scott, 192–93
alpha blockers, 104, 105, 106, 195, 200, 201–2
alpha receptors, 196, 197, 200
ambulatory monitor, 29, 30
Amigo, Isaac, 22
amlodipine (Norvasc), 152, 201, 202
Anderson, Gunnar, 140
anger, 78, 84, 198
angiotensin antagonists, 204, 205, 206, 208, 209 (see also ACE inhibitors)
antianxiety drugs, 104, 106, 116, 178
antidepressant drugs, 104, 105, 106, 116, 130, 178
antihypertensive drugs. See drug therapy
anxiety. See stress and anxiety
anxiety disorder, 127–28
Apresoline (hydralazine), 201
arrhythmias, 120–22, 201
arteries, 12, 15, 137, 197, 198, 205, 206

asthma, 141, 195
atenolol (Tenormin), 106, 121, 152, 200
Ativan (lorazepam), 104
Attwood, Stephen, 194
Australian trial, 25
avoidance. See hidden emotions
awareness, 156–57, 167–68, 219–20, 224

back pain, 117, 156, 176
behavioral/cognitive techniques, 177–78
Benson, Herbert, 37
Berkman, Lisa, 182–83
beta blockers, 104, 105, 106, 152, 195, 200, 201, 202, 204, 205, 206, 209
beta receptors, 197, 198, 203
Bettelheim, Bruno, 73
biofeedback, 37, 177, 192, 215
blood-pressure
    diastolic pressure, 12, 13
    home measurement, 23, 29–30, 137, 142
    measurement, 13, 14
    normal fluctuations, 12–13, 25–26, 32, 199
    normal reading, 12, 29
    physician's attitude and, 27–29
    profile, 30
    reactivity, 32–33
    severity, 139–40
    systolic pressure, 12–13, 19
    temporary elevations, 21–22, 23, 26–27, 32
    time of day, 29
    See also hypertension
blood vessel constriction, 200, 204, 206

238